Laparoscopic Techniques in Uro-Oncology

Laparoscopic Techniques in Uro-Oncology

by

Bertrand Guillonneau, MD
Department of Surgery
Memorial Sloan Kettering Cancer Center
New York, NY, USA

Inderbir S. Gill, MD
Department of Urology, Keck School of Medicine
University of Southern California
Los Angeles, CA, USA

Günter Janetschek, MD
Department of Urology, Paracelsus Medical University
Salzburg, Austria

Ingolf A. Tuerk, MD, PhD
Department of Urology, St. Elizabeth's Medical Center
Boston, MA, USA

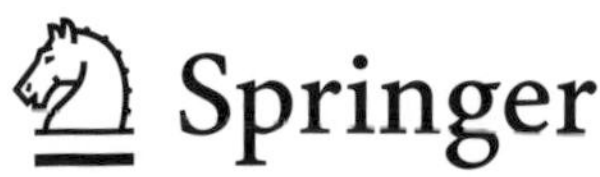

Bertrand Guillonneau, MD
Professor of Urology
Weill Medical College
Cornell University
and
Attending and Head
Section of Minimally Invasive Urology
Memorial Sloan Kettering Cancer Center
New York, NY, USA

Günter Janetschek, MD
Department of Urology
Paracelsus Medical University
Salzburg, Austria

Inderbir S. Gill, MD, MCh
Chairman and The Donald G. Skinner Professor
Department of Urology
Executive Director, USC Institute of Urology
Associate Dean (Clinical Innovation)
Keck School of Medicine
University of Southern California
Los Angeles, CA, USA

Ingolf A. Tuerk, MD, PhD
Professor of Urology
Tufts University
Chief of Urology
St. Elizabeth's Medical Center
Boston, MA, USA

ISBN: 978-1-84628-521-9 e-ISBN: 978-1-84628-789-3
DOI: 10.1007/978-1-84628-789-3

British Library Cataloguing in Publication Data
A catalogue record of this book is available from the British Library

Library of Congress Control Number: 2008944090

Printed on acid-free paper

Springer Science+Business Media
springer.com

Foreword

Laparoscopic surgery, both free-hand and robotic-assisted, has proved to be a transformational technology with a major impact on urologic oncology. While academic urologists today vigorously debate whether a procedure done laparoscopically yields better outcomes than the comparable open procedure, urologic surgeons are voting with their feet: they are performing more and more laparoscopic surgeries every year. The overwhelming interest in laparoscopic surgery is apparent at every urological meeting, but it is perhaps most evident in urologic training programs. Young urologists clearly understand that they must learn minimally invasive techniques if they are to be competitive in practice, particularly in the field of oncology.

Regardless of the outcome of this debate, the development of laparoscopic surgery has wrought a major resurgence of interest in the importance of surgical technique. A decade ago, surgeons themselves seemed bored by presentations or publications that described a surgical technique. There was a general sense that it had all been worked out long ago. That attitude seems oddly out of place today, when our literature and our meetings are filled with intense debates about the differences between surgical approaches and the importance of technique. We now know, for example, that with regard to all important outcomes of major cancer, the skill and experience of the surgeon have a profound impact on the results of surgery. We know that there is a learning curve, sometimes remarkably prolonged, for crucial outcomes such as cancer control after prostatectomy.

Recent studies suggest that both short- and intermediate-term outcomes appear to be comparable between open and some minimally invasive approaches, such as robotic-assisted laparoscopic prostatectomy. Much of this improvement has come from refinements in the open surgical approach to meet the challenge of the laparoscopic approach. When laparoscopic prostatectomy was first performed in 1992, the median hospital stay for patients in the United States after the open procedure was nine days and the median blood loss well over a liter. The typical incision was from the pubis to the umbilicus. Today, in hospitals where robotic surgery has become common, the median length of stay for both robotic and open prostatectomy is the same, less than two days. The need for narcotics, the estimated blood loss, and even the time to convalescence and complete return to normal activities are similar. An analogous story can be told of open surgery for kidney cancer, with the development of increasingly smaller incisions and more conservative surgery. Thus, laparoscopic surgery has had a profound effect on open surgery, constantly pushing open surgeons to develop kinder and gentler techniques while continuing to strive for the best possible long-term outcomes.

Laparoscopic approaches, whether free-hand or robotic-assisted, are radically different from comparable open procedures and call for an entirely different set of skills. One great advantage of this different skill set is that some surgeons who struggled to get good results with the open procedure found that they were highly adept at the laparoscopic or robotic-assisted procedures. Of course, others found the new techniques challenging and did not adopt them. While laparoscopic surgery may not be the right tool for every surgeon, our patients benefit from having access to a variety of approaches that can achieve good results.

One worries about the intoxicating effects of dazzling new technology. While the da Vinci robot is a remarkably complex and sophisticated machine, it has proven disappointing by not giving us better overall long-term results than can be achieved with good open surgery. This does not mean that the surgical robot is a distraction or an unnecessary expense, but that the capability of the current robot may not offer sufficient advantages over open surgical techniques to overcome the limitations of inflexibility, loss of haptic feedback, and loss of direct visualization of the field.

There is every reason to be optimistic about the future of laparoscopic surgery, whether free-hand or robotic. This approach can readily incorporate modern technological breakthroughs that would prove difficult during open surgery. One excellent example is the possibility of the "glowing margin," in which a monoclonal antibody to prostate cancer, labeled with a fluorophore, could be given to the patient a day before the operation. Then, during laparoscopic prostatectomy, a laser built in to the camera system could flash for a few milliseconds and create a readily visible glow in the area of cancer. This kind of technology is readily adaptable to the bloodless field and camera system inherent in laparoscopic surgery.

Laparoscopic Techniques in Uro-Oncology is an enormously valuable educational tool for young surgeons learning these techniques for the first time, as well as for established surgeons constantly seeking to improve. Written by four giants in the field, representing both the European and American developments in laparoscopic surgery, this beautifully illustrated book provides not only fundamental insight into the laparoscopic anatomy of the genitourinary system but also details numerous tricks of the trade that can lead to improved techniques and better results. The authors are to be congratulated on a monumental task. They challenged themselves to produce a text that would teach surgical technique, and they have succeeded remarkably well. It is hard to imagine how any serious surgeon performing laparoscopic surgery for a genitourinary cancer would be comfortable without having this text readily at hand. I can imagine seeing it in the operating room, in conference rooms, and in the offices of every urologic cancer surgeon. It is a wonderful, lucid, and highly effective compilation of surgical insights from the most brilliant leaders in the field.

One already hopes that future editions will be produced on a regular basis, incorporating the authors' insights in this rapidly evolving field.

Peter T. Scardino, MD
Chairman, Department of Surgery
Memorial Sloan-Kettering Cancer Center
David H. Koch Chair

Preface

Since its introduction more than 15 years ago, urologic laparoscopy has matured significantly, emerging as a sound, viable alternative for many patients with renal, testicular, bladder, prostate and other urologic cancers. In recent times we have witnessed the emergence of the discipline of minimally invasive uro-oncology and advanced minimally invasive surgical techniques are now a strong viable partner to radical open surgery.

This is a "technique" book intended for urologists with prior experience in basic laparoscopy and uro-oncology. The focus is on practical, step-by-step details and subtleties. We have intentionally omitted any discussion of diagnoses, indications, instrumentation, or basics of laparoscopic access; there are already excellent textbooks dealing with these issues. The techniques we have described here are based on the aggregate of our personal experiences performing over 8,000 laparoscopic surgeries. We have tried to distill "what works" based on our knowledge of the errors made and the successes that have withstood the test of time. Not all techniques are described, and many variants are omitted. This does not mean those techniques have no value, but rather that we prefer the ones presented herein.

We hope this book will assist laparoscopic urologic oncologists in offering their patients a technically superior operation, performed in the safest manner. If this is the case, our work of the past 15 years would be validated. For the four of us, it has been a true privilege to participate in the development of this field and it is equally gratifying for us to share our collective experience with our colleagues.

Bertrand Guillonneau
Inderbir S. Gill
Günter Janetschek
Ingolf A. Tuerk

Acknowledgments

A book is not made by one, two, or even four writers. It is a formidable project that involves many other people who contribute their knowledge, skills, and practical experience. In a technical textbook such as this, surgeons have the most visible place. But beyond the four named authors, this book has been brought to fruition by many more. They should be thanked here for their insights, critiques, comments, and support during the development of this textbook. It would be impossible to thank all of them in this space and we apologize to them in advance for these omissions.

We would like also to thank urology editorial team at Memorial Sloan-Kettering Cancer Center: Susan Aiello, Barbara Kristaponis, Michael McGregor, Peggy McPartland, Janet Novak, and Joyce Tsoi for their help in the effort to make this information clear and understandable. We would like, in addition, to acknowledge Melissa Morton at Springer for her enthusiastic support and for her patience. Springer has trusted us and allowed us to bring to the urological community this sum of our experience.

If this textbook meets the expectation of our peers and is useful to future laparoscopic surgeons, it is because all of these endeavors were indispensable.

We would like to extend special acknowledgment to the following physicians and surgeons:

Nadcem Abu-Rustum
Memorial Sloan Kettering Cancer Center, New York, NY, USA
Nasser Albqami, MD
Hospital of the Elisabethinen, Linz, Austria
Monish Aron, MD
Cleveland Clinic Foundation, Cleveland, Ohio, USA
David Canes, MD
Lahey Clinic Medical Center, Burlington, Massachusetts, USA
Xavier Cathelineau, MD
Institut Mutualiste Montsouris, Paris, France
Mihir Desai, MD
Cleveland Clinic Foundation, Cleveland, Ohio, USA
Georges-Pascal Haber, MD
Cleveland Clinic Foundation, Cleveland, Ohio, USA
Jihad Kaouk, MD
Cleveland Clinic Foundation, Cleveland, Ohio, USA

John A. Libertino, MD
Chairman
Lahey Clinic Institute of Urology
Lahey Clinic Medical Center, Burlington, Massachusetts, USA
Andrew C. Novick, MD
Chairman
Glickman Urological and Kidney Institute
Cleveland Clinic Foundation, Cleveland, Ohio, USA
Peter T. Scardino, MD
Chairman
Department of Surgery
Memorial Sloan-Kettering Cancer Center, New York, New York, USA
Fernando P. Secin, MD, PhD
Instituto Universitario–Centro de Educación Médica e Investigaciones Clínicas,
Buenos Aires, Argentina
Andrea Sorcini, MD
Lahey Clinic Medical Center, Burlington, Massachusetts, USA
A. Karim Touijer, MD
Memorial Sloan-Kettering Cancer Center, New York, New York, USA
Guy Vallancien
Chairman, Department of Urology, Institut Mutualiste Montsouris, Paris, France

Contents

1 Laparoscopic Anatomy of the Upper Urinary Tract: Intra-Abdominal and Retroperitoneal Approaches

Laparoscopy, with its advantages and limitations, requires a different topographic comprehension of surgical anatomy, adapted to a certain angle of vision and magnification. The anatomical perspective of the surgical field during laparoscopy is somewhat different from that usually seen during open surgery, and considering the anatomy from a different perspective is a prerequisite for performing safe and efficient surgery. Therefore, mastering laparoscopic topographic anatomy becomes indispensable for identifying structures and recognizing their spatial relationships. This chapter presents the topographic anatomy of the retroperitoneum as it appears to the laparoscopist. Positional relationships follow standard anatomical terminology, so that superior, inferior, anterior, and posterior refer to positions toward the head, feet, surface, and back, respectively. The right and left upper urinary tracts are presented separately.

For transperitoneal laparoscopy of the upper abdomen, the patient is placed on the operating table in a 45° lateral decubitus position, and the table is slightly flexed. For retroperitoneal laparoscopy, the patient is placed in a 90° standard flank position.

Right Upper Urinary Tract

Intra-Abdominal Approach

During transperitoneal laparoscopy, the anatomy can be seen clearly as soon as the laparoscope is introduced into the abdominal cavity. The liver lies on the organs of the upper retroperitoneum (Figure 1.1) and so must always be retracted to gain access to the adrenal gland and the upper pole of the kidney. The gallbladder comes into view when the liver is lifted up. The hepatoduodenal ligament travels between the dorsal aspect of the

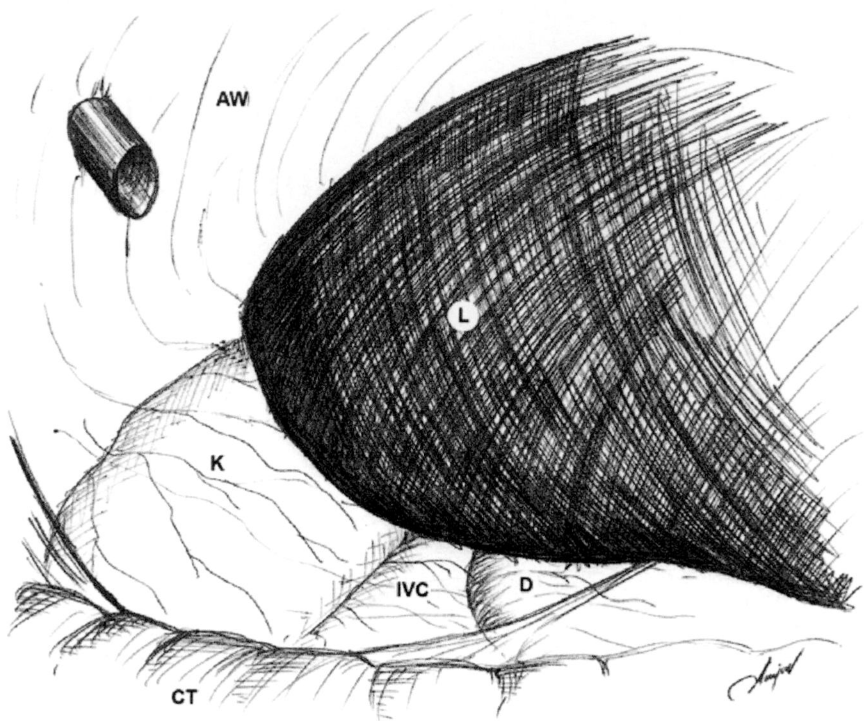

FIGURE 1.1. View of upper right abdomen (laparoscope in umbilicus, 30° lens). AW = lateral abdominal wall, CT = transverse colon, D = duodenum, IVC = inferior vena cava, K = kidney, L = liver

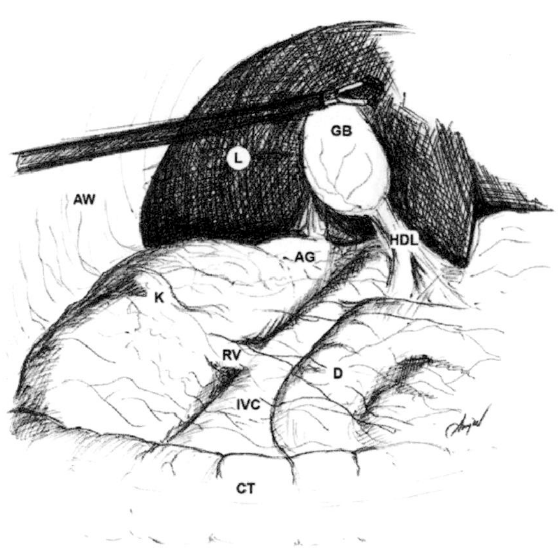

FIGURE 1.2. View of upper right abdomen after retraction of liver. AG = adrenal gland, AW = lateral abdominal wall, CT = transverse colon, D = duodenum, GB = gallbladder, HDL = hepatoduodenal ligament, IVC = inferior vena cava, K = kidney, L = liver, RV = renal vein

liver and the duodenum. The entrance into the bursa omentalis is between the hepatoduodenic ligament and the inferior vena cava (Figure 1.2). The cecum, ascending colon, right colonic flexure, and transverse colon are always visible, even in obese patients.

The lower pole of the right kidney and the proximal ureter are covered by the colonic flexure and the transverse colon. Most of the right kidney, however, can be considered as "intra-abdominal" and is covered only by Gerota's fascia and the peritoneum (Figures 1.1 and 1.2). The same is true of the right adrenal gland, which lies directly underneath and posterior to the peritoneum (Figure 1.2). At the level of the renal veins, the ventral surface of the inferior vena cava is covered by the transverse colon and duodenum. Its caudal portion disappears underneath the transverse colon (Figures 1.2 and 1,3). Cranial to the duodenum, the vena cava is covered only by the peritoneum, and it can be recognized before any dissection in thin patients (Figure 1.2). See Figure 1.3 for anatomy of

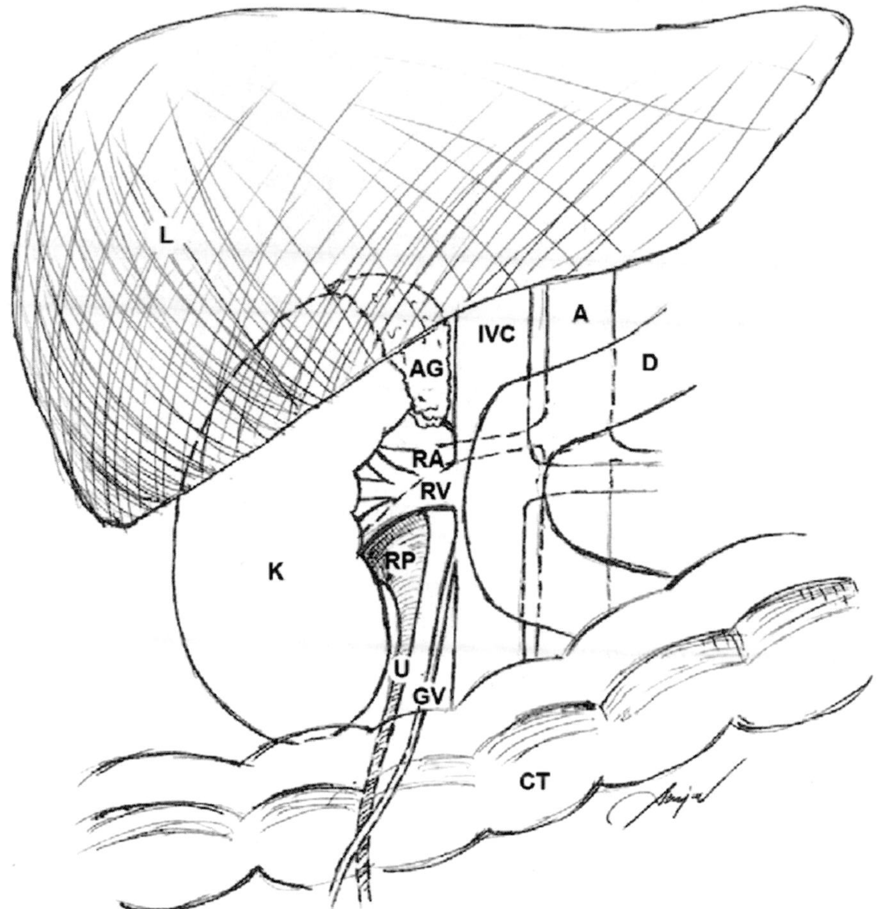

FIGURE 1.3. Anatomy of upper right abdomen. Figure key: A = aorta, AG = adrenal gland, CT = transverse colon, D = duodenum, GV = gonadal vessel, IVC = inferior vena cava, K = kidney, L = liver, RA = renal artery, RP = renal pelvis, RV = renal vein, U = ureter

the kidney, its vessels, and the ureter in relation to the surrounding structures.

Exposure of the Retroperitoneum

Complete exposure of the retroperitoneum requires dissection of the ascending colon and the right colonic flexure in the plane of Toldt's fascia. During displacement of the transverse colon, care must be taken with the lower part of the duodenum, which crosses just dorsal to the colon. The duodenum and the head of the pancreas are then displaced medially, and the retroperitoneum becomes freely accessible (Figure 1.4). The extent of dissection of the bowel, however, depends largely on the procedure that is to be done. Adrenalectomy, for example, requires only retraction of the liver, with no dissection of the colon and no or only minimal dissection of the duodenum. For radical nephrectomy, minimal displacement of the transverse colon and right colonic flexure is required, but some dissection of the duodenum is necessary to expose the right renal pedicle. In contrast, retroperitoneal lymph node dissection for testicular cancer requires wide exposure of the entire retroperitoneum, because the interaortocaval space has to be approached as well. This can be achieved only after complete medial displacement of the entire right colon, the duodenum, and the head of the pancreas.

Kidney, Ureter, and Renal Vessels

After exposure of the retroperitoneum in the plane of Toldt's fascia, the right renal vein is readily accessible (Figure 1.4). The key landmark for

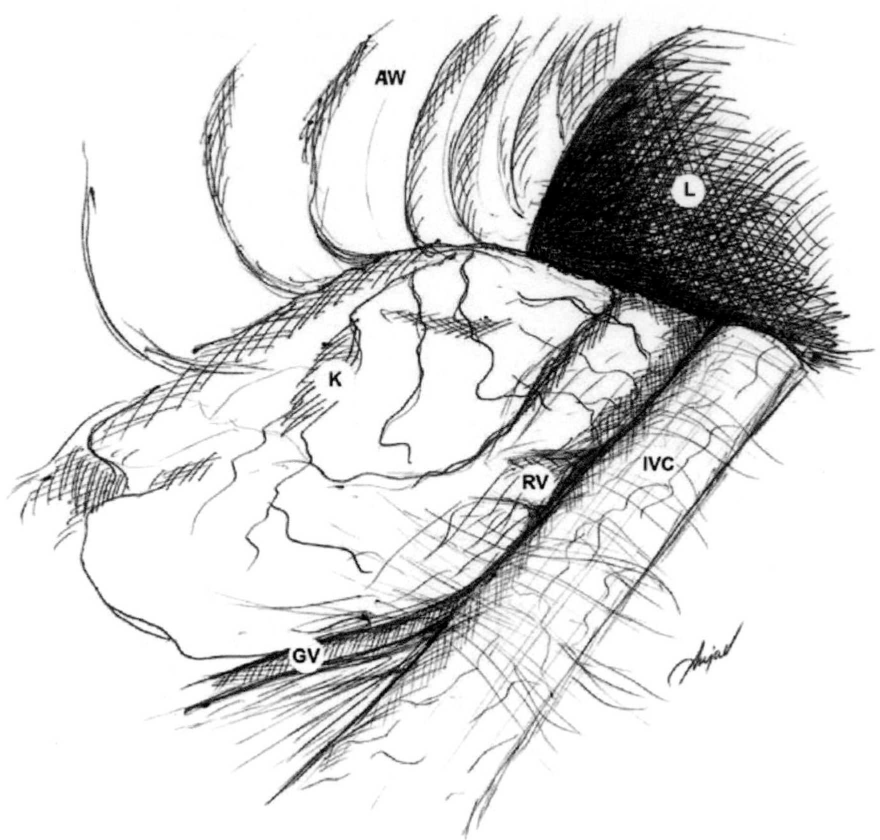

FIGURE 1.4. View of upper right abdomen after medial displacement of colon and duodenum and retraction of liver. AW = lateral abdominal wall, GV = gonadal vessel, IVC = inferior vena cava, K = kidney, L = liver, RV = renal vein

the approach to the right ureter is the gonadal vein. It opens into the inferior vena cava a few centimeters below the right renal vein. The retroperitoneum is opened on the lateral edge of the gonadal vein. Dissection is performed down to the psoas muscle. Further caudal dissection reveals the ureter, which crosses the gonadal vein on its dorsal side (Figure 1.3). In the area of the crossing, several venous anastomoses between the gonadal and ureteral veins require careful dissection and meticulous hemostasis. Cranial to the crossing, the ureter is lateral to the gonadal vein; while caudal to the crossing, the ureter runs medial to the gonadal vein. It is important to remember the ventrodorsal orientation of structures at the crossing: gonadal vein <n> ureter <n> psoas muscle. To approach the renal artery (e.g., for a nephrectomy), the lower pole of the kidney must be freed and lifted up (Figure 1.3).

Caveats: Although the gonadal vein typically inserts into the inferior vena cava, it can insert into the right renal vein as well. If this potential anomalous relationship is not recognized, the renal vein can initially be confused with the inferior vena cava and be a source of serious iatrogenic injury. Such anomalous vasculature (among other things) can be identified by a preoperative 3-D CT scan. Accessory renal blood vessels may or may not lie in a slightly more anterior plane than the main renal vessels and are end arteries without collateral supply. As a rule, the right inferior polar artery is always precaval. Such accessory renal arteries and the often accompanying accessory renal vein are present in approximately 20% of patients.

Adrenal Gland

A specific understanding of adrenal surgical anatomy is key for the safe performance of laparoscopic adrenalectomy. Located within the retroperitoneum and inside Gerota's fascia, the adrenal glands are separated from the upper pole of the kidney by a fibrous layer. Both adrenal glands are distinct in shape and size, anatomic location and relationships with adjacent structures, and vascular supply.

The triangular-shaped right adrenal gland lies cranial and slightly medial to the superior pole of the kidney. The right adrenal gland is the most superior organ structure in the right half of the retroperitoneum. As such, accessing the right adrenal gland during transperitoneal laparoscopy requires that the liver is substantially retracted superiorly. The medial portion of the adrenal gland abuts the inferior vena cava and, at times, a significant portion of its parenchyma can be located retrocaval (posterior to the inferior vena cava).

Superiorly, the adrenal gland abuts the under surface of the liver. Laterally, the adrenal gland is bounded by the most inferior portions of the diaphragm and the lateral abdominal wall. Posteriorly, the adrenal gland lies atop the psoas muscle and receives collateral blood supply from small arterial perforating vessels originating from the inferior phrenic artery (superior pedicle), the aorta (middle pedicle), and the right renal artery (inferior pedicle). Specific and identifiable arteries to the adrenal gland usually cannot be discretely identified. However, a single, short adrenal vein drains directly into the inferior vena cava. This adrenal vein is a short, wide vessel, originating from the superior-medial aspect of the adrenal gland, that enters directly into the lateral aspect of the inferior vena cava in a high infrahepatic location. This means that the adrenal vein cannot be seen without significant cranial mobilization of the liver. Identifying the adrenal vein is strongly recommended before making any attempt to mobilize the adrenal gland. If the vein tears, it will avulse at its junction into the inferior vena cava, which can lead to significant bleeding that is difficult to control.

Retroperitoneal Approach

Kidney

After the surgeon has obtained proper retroperitoneal access, the psoas muscle becomes the horizontal floor of the surgeon's view and his or her main landmark throughout the surgery. This horizontal orientation must be maintained at all times (Figure 1.5). To see the bulk of the kidney and to be able to apply

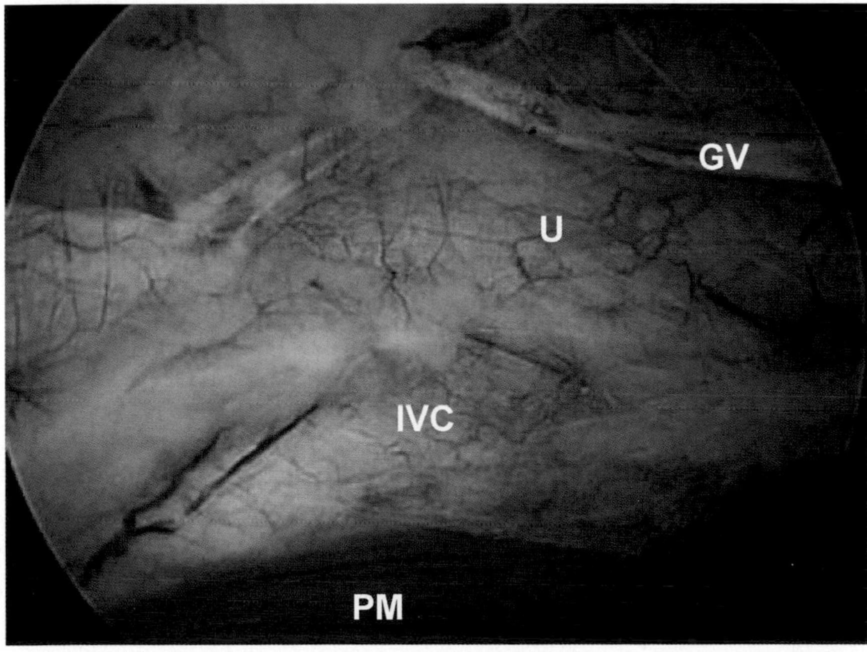

FIGURE 1.5. Right retroperitoneal approach: psoas muscle (PM), inferior vena cava (IVC), ureter (U), gonadal vessel (GV)

adequate anterior traction on the kidney, it is necessary to identify the bands that attach Gerota's fascia to the psoas fascia. These bands must initially be incised sharply, followed by blunt dissection to separate the kidney and associated Gerota's fascia from the fascia of the psoas muscle. The main renal blood vessels can be seen when the laparoscope is at a 45° angle to the body's horizon. The pulsations of the renal artery can be detected in this view. In this retroperitoneal approach, the renal vein, anterior to the renal artery, cannot be fully visualized until the renal artery has been completely dissected (Figure 1.6).

After the renal artery has been divided, the renal vein is seen more medially and anterior (or superiorly according to the surgeon's perspective). In this same perspective, the ureter is seen just anterior to (above) the inferior vena cava, and the gonadal vein is seen further anterior to the ureter (Figure 1.7). The kidney and associated Gerota's fascia can be dissected sharply from the peritoneum by incising the thin, bloodless areolar tissue between them.

Caveats: The gently undulating pulsations of the inferior vena cava should be identified early in the surgery. If the inferior vena cava is not clearly identified, dissection can be done inadvertently posterior, in a retrocaval fashion. Inadvertent transection of the inferior vena cava in the retroperitoneal approach has been reported (as it has in the transperitoneal approach). The three sentinel guidelines for avoiding this complication are 1) to identify the cranial and caudal right angle junction of the right renal vein to the inferior vena cava, 2) to ensure the camera is properly oriented by seeing the psoas muscle as the horizonal horizon, and 3) to visualize the renal vein coursing toward the kidney (superior, according to the surgeon's perspective).

Adrenal Gland

Right retroperitoneal laparoscopic adrenal surgery has three anatomically related major advantages over traditional open adrenal surgery: there is no requirement for bowel and liver mobilization, the adrenal vein can be rapidly identified and controlled, and direct access to any retrocaval portion of the adrenal gland ensures complete resection in case of cancer surgery.

The right adrenal vein is best approached by first identifying the location of the hilum of the right kidney (as described above) (see Figures 1.8 and

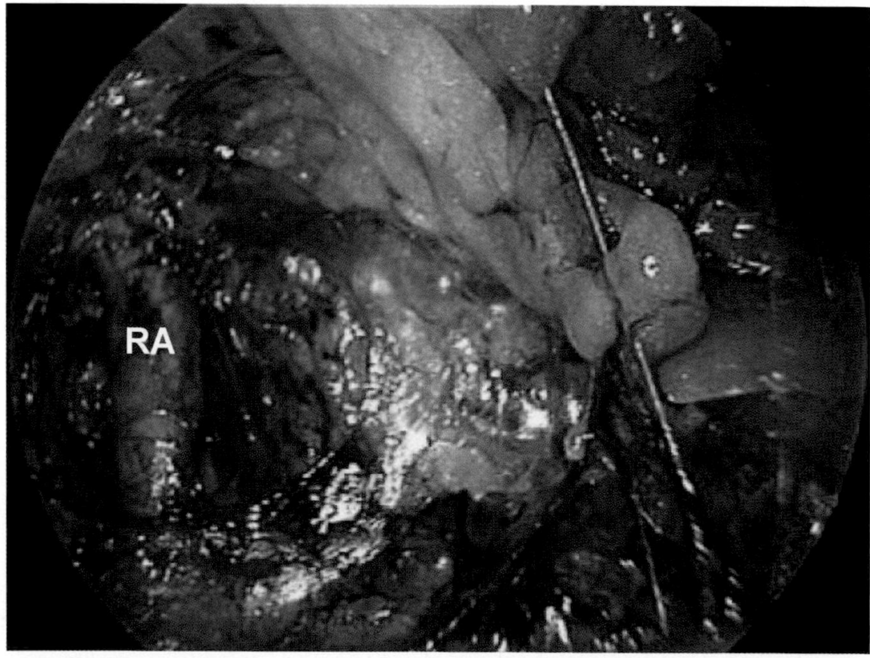

FIGURE 1.6. Right retroperitoneal approach: renal artery (RA) located vertical and posterior, after incision of Gerota's fascia posteriorly

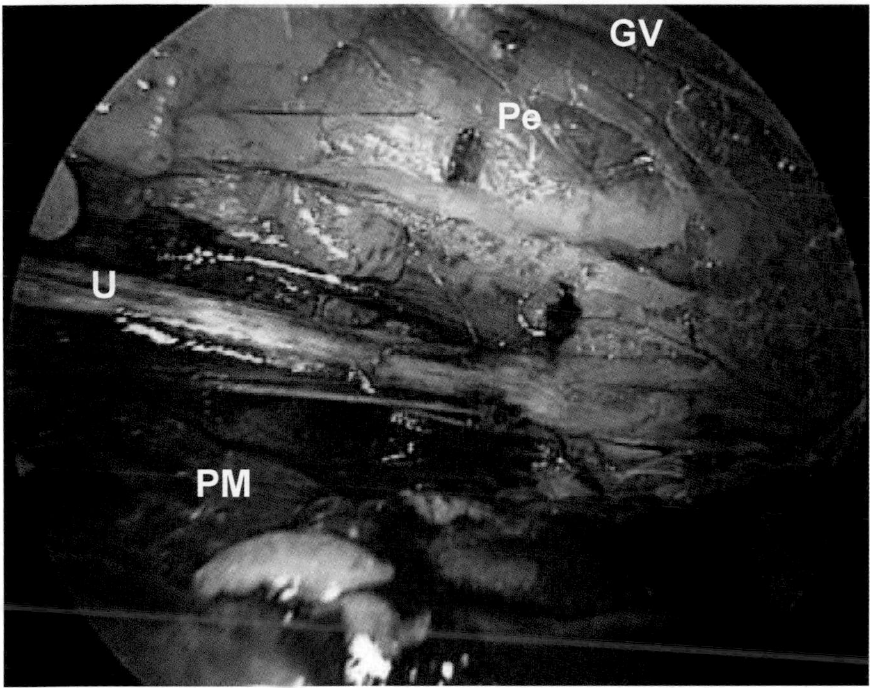

FIGURE 1.7. Right retroperitoneal approach: ureter (U) located under peritoneum (Pe) and anterior to psoas muscle (PM); gonadal vessel (GV) located above ureter

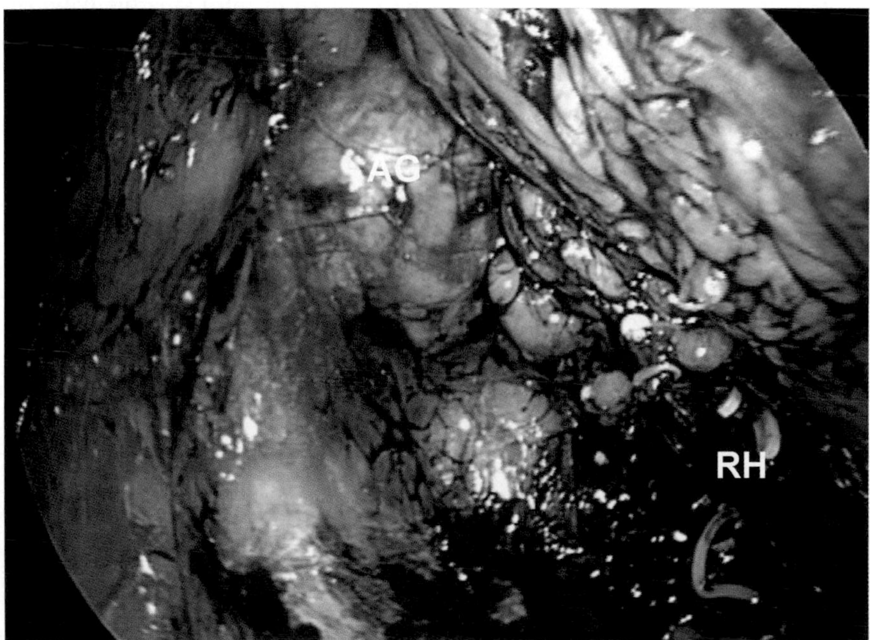

FIGURE 1.8. Right retroperitoneal approach: After Gerota's fascia has been opened, kidney should be lifted up and renal hilum (RH) dissected to isolate adrenal gland (AG) at upper pole of kidney

3.17). Dissection immediately superior to the right renal vein and directly along the inferior vena cava in a cranial direction will bring the adrenal vein into view (Figure 3.18). The inferior vena cava acts as "the guide to the right adrenal vein," which in this retroperitoneal approach, is usually seen coursing anterior and medially when anterior traction is applied to the adrenal gland. Of course, the direction in which the adrenal vein is seen depends entirely on the angle at which the surgeon applies traction to the adrenal gland. As is the case for the renal vein, the cranial and caudal junctions of the adrenal vein to the inferior vena cava must be seen before ligating the adrenal vein. Dissection far cranially on the inferior vena cava, superior to the adrenal vein, would reveal the hepatic veins.

Cranially, the adrenal gland is also held to the peritoneum by some attachments that need to be freed, while anteriorly the gland is typically separated from the peritoneum only by a bloodless, areolar tissue. Inferiorly, the dissection of the adrenal gland leaves the superior pole of the right kidney bare.

Caveats: After traction has been applied to the adrenal gland and before the adrenal vein has been ligated and transected, the inferior vena cava may be kinked and not course in the expected direction cranial to the adrenal vein.

If overzealous dissection is performed too far cranially along the inferior vena cava, the hepatic veins may be encountered. When possible, freeing the caudal attachments of the adrenal gland to the kidney should be the last step in adrenal gland mobilization. This is beneficial because once Gerota's fascia is entered, a significant amount of unwieldy perirenal fat narrows the surgeon's field of view.

Left Upper Urinary Tract

Intra-Abdominal Approach

In contrast to the right kidney, the left kidney appears completely retroperitoneal. It is covered by the left colonic flexure and spleen. Compared with the right colonic flexure, the left flexure is more cranial, at the level of the renal vessels or even more superior (Figure 1.9). The left colonic flexure is fixed to the lateral abdominal wall by a fibrous ligament (Figure 1.10) and connected to the caudal surface of the spleen by the splenocolic ligament, in which several thin-walled veins are present. Therefore, incising or transecting the ligament must be done carefully. The upper pole of the kidney and the adrenal gland are covered by the spleen (Figures 1.9 and 1.10). Ventral to the adrenal gland, the tail of the pancreas is in contact with the spleen (Figure 1.9).

Exposure of the Retroperitoneum

Complete exposure of the retroperitoneum requires medial displacement of the left colonic flexure, the descending colon, and the spleen. For exposure of the lower retroperitoneum, displacement of the descending colon is sufficient.

Displacement of the colon: Dissection is started caudally at the level of the pelvic brim by incising the line of Toldt lateral to the colon. This incision is continued cranially toward the colonic flexure. The fibrous attachments of the flexure are cut close to the abdominal wall. The colon and its mesentery are released from the retroperitoneum in the almost avascular plane of Toldt. The colonic flexure, which is in close contact with Gerota's fascia of the lower pole, must be approached carefully. It can be tempting to continue dissection in a wrong plane between Gerota's fascia and the lateral abdominal wall instead of separating the two layers. The ventral surface of Gerota's fascia must be dissected free completely, exposing the proximal ureter and pelvis. Incising or transecting the splenocolic ligament improves exposure of the renal hilum. Making this incision close to the spleen allows for better control of the veins within the ligament and for separation of the transverse colon from the spleen and the tail of the pancreas. Retroperitoneal lymph node dissection for testicular cancer requires complete medial displacement of the bowel, but no additional dissection of the spleen.

Displacement of the colon and spleen: Dissection is started as described above in the line of Toldt, lateral to the colon. After the surgeon has released the colonic flexure from the abdominal wall, dissection is continued cranially by incising the peritoneum lateral to the spleen (Figure 1.11). This incision is continued all the way to the diaphragm. In addition to the medial displacement of the colon (as described above), the spleen and especially the tail of the pancreas are released from Gerota's fascia of the upper pole and from the ventral surface of the adrenal gland. As a result of this dissection, the spleen can

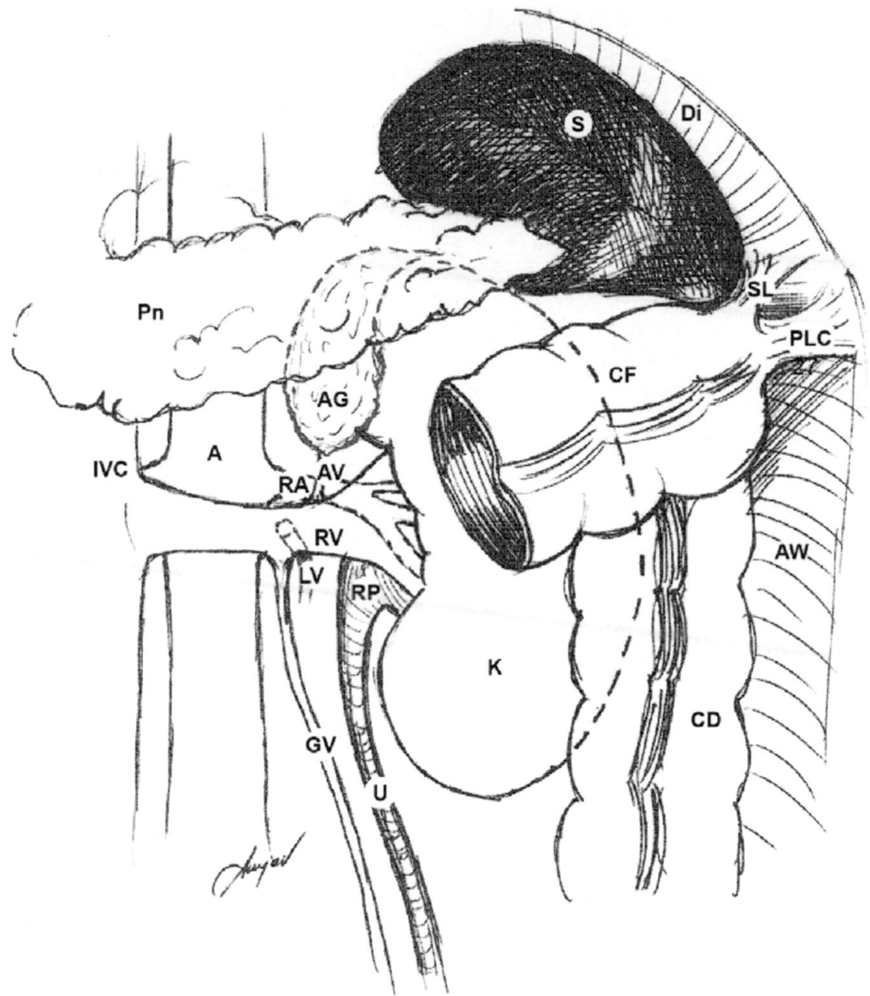

FIGURE 1.9. View of upper left abdomen (laparoscope in umbilicus, 30° lens). A = aorta, AG = adrenal gland, AV = adrenal vein, AW = lateral abdominal wall, CD = descending colon, CF = colonic flexure, Di = diaphragm, GV = gonadal vessel, IVC = inferior vena cava, K = kidney, LV = lumbar vein, PCL = phrenocolonic ligament, Pn = pancreas, RA = renal artery, RP = renal pelvis, RV = renal vein, S = spleen, SL = splenocolonic ligament, U = ureter

be rotated medially about 180° so that the entire upper retroperitoneum becomes freely accessible (Figure 1.12). Incising the splenocolic ligament is usually not necessary but may improve exposure in some patients. For adrenalectomy, complete dissection of the spleen is particularly advantageous, while dissection of the colon can be limited.

Kidney, Ureter, and Renal Vessels

Anatomy of the left side of the retroperitoneum differs in some details from that of the right side. Identifying the left renal vein is usually more difficult. It may therefore be helpful to first identify the gonadal vein, which can be followed cranially where it opens into the renal vein. The adrenal vein enters the renal vein at its cranial border and medial to the gonadal vein. Frequently, a lumbar vein can be seen entering the renal vein on its dorsal side (Figure 1.9). Because this lumbar vein travels caudal to the renal artery, the artery can be approached only after the lumbar vein has been transected. Early transection of the adrenal vein is easy when required, for instance, for a pheochromocytoma.

The relationship between the gonadal vein and the ureter on the left side is similar to that on the right

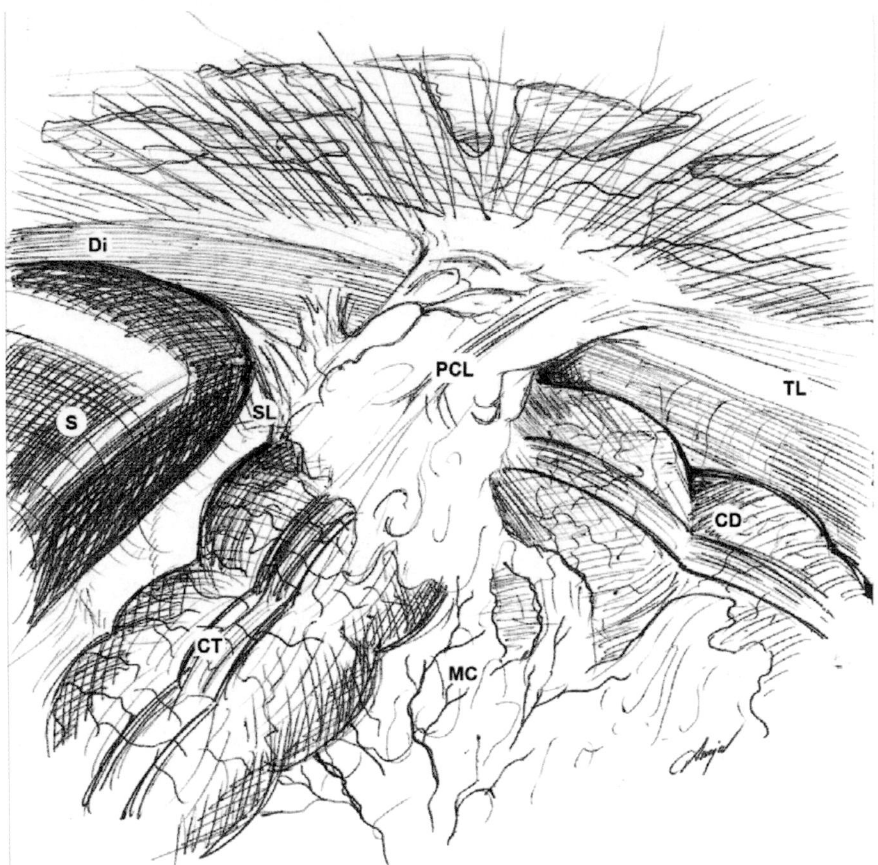

FIGURE 1.10. Anatomy of upper left abdomen. CD = descending colon, CT = transverse colon, Di = diaphragm, MC = mesocolon, SL = splenocolonic ligament, PCL = phrenocolonic ligament, S = spleen, TL = line of Toldt

side, and they cross at the same level. Therefore, the gonadal vein can be used as a landmark to approach the ureter. For a nephrectomy, however, the retroperitoneum is entered medial (not lateral) to the gonadal vein, which directly enters the renal vein on the left side. Therefore, the cranial portion of the vein is removed along with the kidney.

Transmesenteric Approach to the Renal Hilum

As in open surgery, the renal hilum can be approached directly by incising the peritoneum at the ligament of Treitz (duodenojejunal flexure) (Figure1.13). This approach is not recommended in obese patients. The colon is retracted laterally to allow for good exposure. Starting at the ligament of Treitz, the peritoneum is incised at the root of the mesentery of the colon dorsal and parallel to the inferior mesenteric vein in a caudal direction (Figure 1.14). Little dissection is required to identify the ventral surface of the aorta and the caudal edge of the left renal vein. The aorta is followed cranially at its left lateral side to identify the origin of the left renal artery, which can then be ligated safely in a nephrectomy.

Caveats: Placing a nasogastric tube can keep the stomach decompressed. Although uncommon, the body of the stomach can lie just cranial to the upper pole of the left kidney.

The lumbar vein runs directly posterior from the posterior surface of the left renal vein. When this lumbar vein must be specifically identified, such as during a laparoscopic donor nephrectomy, placing

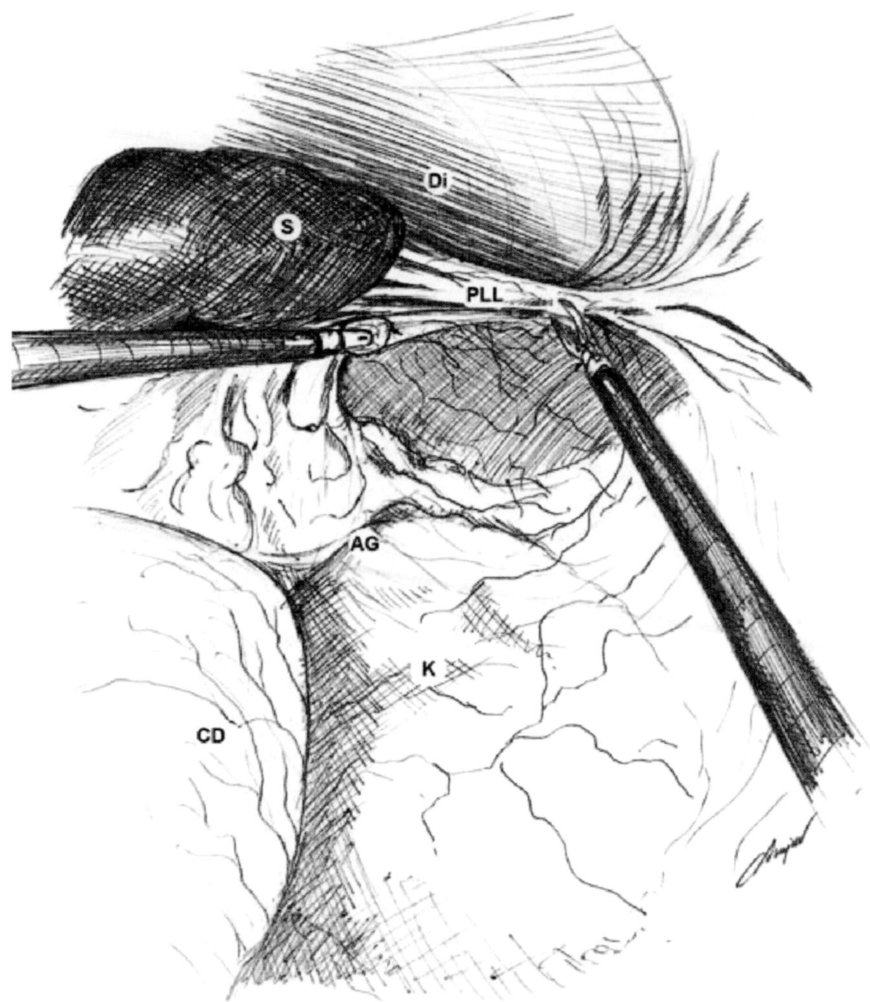

FIGURE 1.11. Upper left abdomen: incision of peritoneum lateral to spleen. AG = adrenal gland, CD = descending colon, Di = diaphragm, PLL = phrenicolienal ligament, K = kidney, S = spleen

a locking clip on the gonadal vein, leaving approximately a 2-cm stump of the gonadal vein attached to the renal vein, is recommended. This stump can then serve as a handle to apply anterior traction on or mobilization of the renal vein, revealing its posterior aspect and, therefore, the lumbar vein (and potentially its branches).

Adrenal Gland

The left adrenal gland, like the right adrenal gland, lies cranial to the upper pole of the kidney. However, unlike the right adrenal gland, the crescent-shaped left adrenal gland lies in a more medial position with respect to the upper pole of the kidney, occupying a lower anatomic position in the retroperitoneum than the right adrenal gland.

Medially, just as the right adrenal gland lies contiguous with the inferior vena cava, the left adrenal gland lies in close proximity to the left lateral boarder of the aorta. Typically, the clearance between the aorta and the left adrenal gland is greater than that between the inferior vena cava and the right adrenal gland, and can be easily demonstrated by a clear fat plane between the aorta and adrenal gland on preoperative 3-D CT scanning.

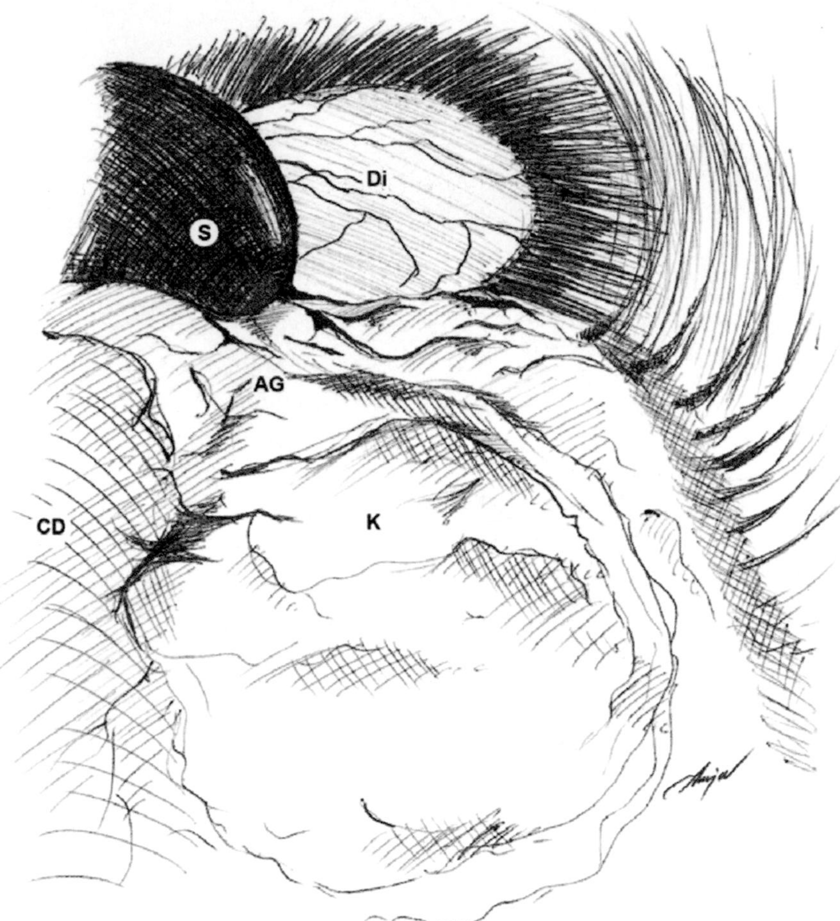

FIGURE 1.12. View of upper left abdomen after medial displacement of colon and spleen.AG = adrenal gland, CD = descending colon, Di = diaphragm, K = kidney, S = spleen

Additionally, on the left side, the adrenal gland does not have a retroaortic portion, while on the right side, the gland often has a retrocaval portion.

Superiorly, the adrenal gland abuts the under surface of the spleen, and inferiorly, the pancreatic tail. Laterally, it is bounded by the most inferior portions of the diaphragm and the pleura and by the lateral abdominal wall. Posteriorly, it lies atop the psoas muscle.

Like that to the right adrenal gland, the blood supply to the left adrenal gland consists of branches of the inferior phrenic artery, the left renal artery, and perforating branches of the aorta. Again, these named arteries are rarely specifically identified.

In contrast to the right adrenal vein, the left main adrenal vein arises from the inferior-medial aspect of the left adrenal gland. The left adrenal vein is narrower and longer, draining into the medial half of the left renal vein in a more medial position relative to the gonadal and lumbar veins. The adrenal vein is visualized by partially dissecting the renal vein. When the renal vein is dissected medially, the insertion of the adrenal vein is seen on the cranial margin of the renal vein.

Caveats: The anteromedial part of the adrenal gland lies very close to the tail of the pancreas. If this relationship is not remembered and if the tail of the pancreas is prominent, the adrenal gland can easily be confused with the tail of the pancreas on initial dissection.

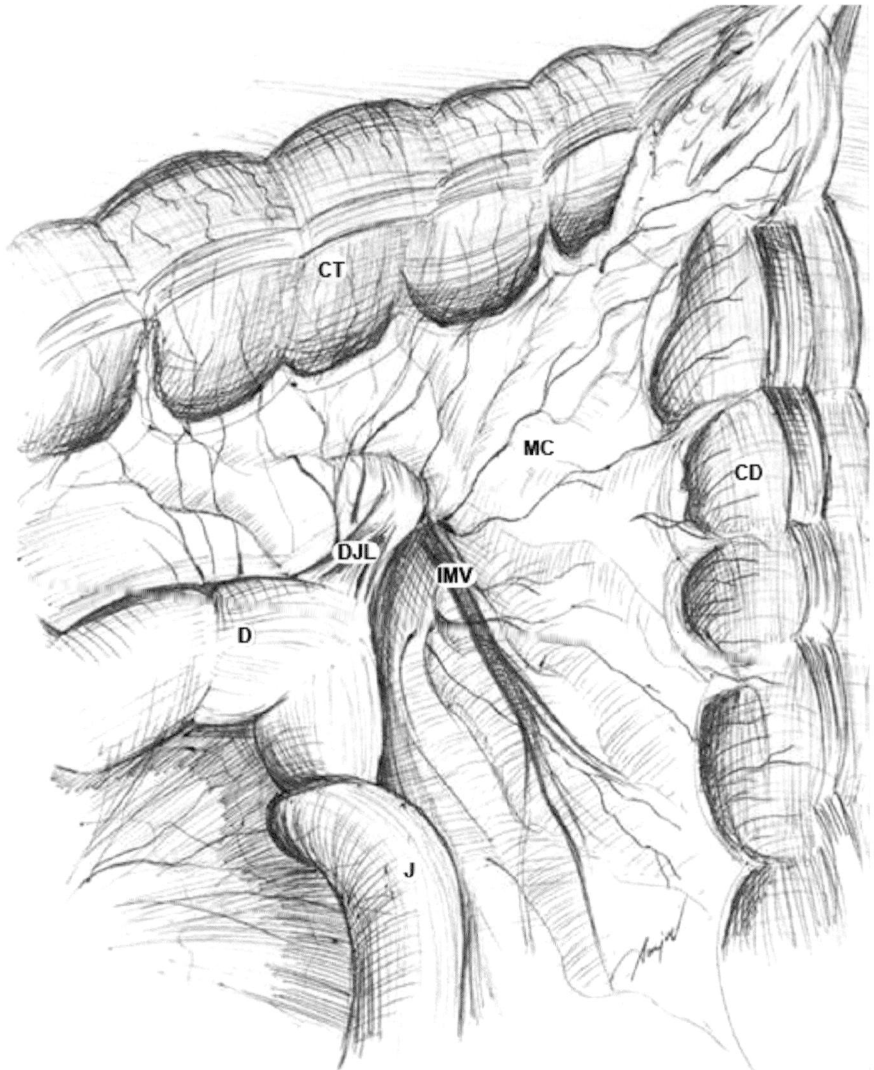

FIGURE 1.13. Transmesenteric approach: exposure before peritoneal incision. D = duodenum, CD = descending colon, CT = transverse colon, DJL =Treitz ligament (duodenojejunic ligament), IMV = inferior mesenteric vein, J = jejunum, MC = mesocolon

Retroperitoneal Approach

Kidney

The retroperitoneal approach to the left kidney differs from that of the right kidney in several critical aspects. First the aorta, rather than the inferior vena cava, is the horizontally running major vessel. Its sharp, horizontal pulsations are easily recognized when the kidney is lifted anteriorly away from the psoas muscle. Although the renal artery pulsations are again seen when the laparoscope is at a 45° angle to the body, in the retroperitoneal view, the surgeon sees the renal artery lying superior (to the right on the monitor) and slightly posterior to the renal vein. On the left side, the renal vein and artery can be seen at the same time running parallel to one another. Additionally on the left side, the level at which the renal vein is ligated and transected is

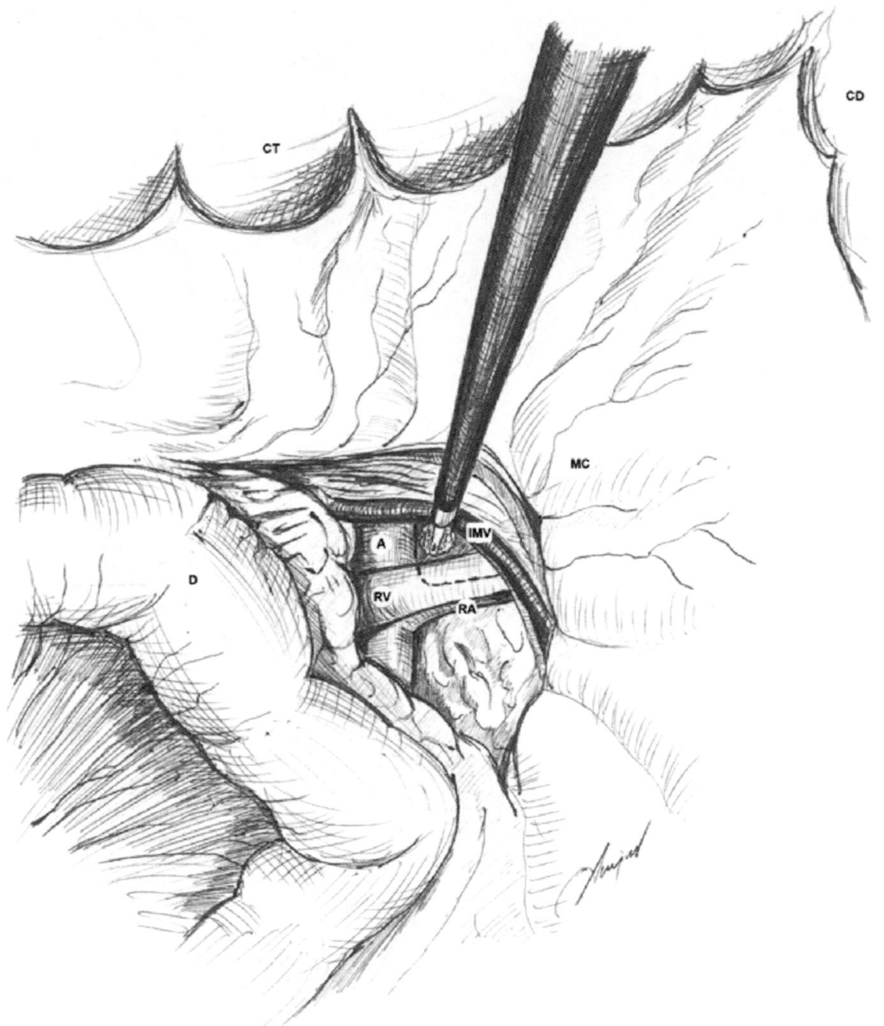

FIGURE 1.14. Transmesenteric approach: dissection of aorta, renal artery, and renal vein. A = aorta, CD = descending colon, CT = transverse colon, D = duodenum, IMV = inferior mesenteric vein, MC = mesocolon, RA = renal artery, RV = renal vein

more lateral (toward the kidney parenchyma) than on the right side. As a result, the adrenal vein usually enters the renal vein medial to where the renal vein has been ligated. This has consequences when performing an adrenalectomy with the nephrectomy (see LEFT UPPER URINARY TRACT, RETROPERITONEAL APPROACH, ADRENAL GLAND, below).

Caveats: At times, a lumbar vein can be seen in the retroperitoneal approach, and it should be ligated after the renal artery has been ligated and transected. This frees the renal vein, facilitating further renal vein dissection. Although it is rare and difficult to visualize the superior mesenteric artery in the retroperitoneal approach, the surgeon must be ever mindful of its anatomic location to avoid iatrogenic injury. The superior mesenteric artery runs anterior to the aorta and medial to the renal artery. Therefore, dissection medial to the renal artery and vein should not be done without being aware of the presence of the root of the superior mesenteric artery. The approach to the medial attachments of the kidney to the aorta or posterior peritoneum should be anterior and lateral (ie, over rather than under the kidney). This enables the surgeon to identify the attachments that are running exclusively *to* the kidney and thereby avoid the superior mesenteric artery. The same principle holds true for left adrenal gland dissection.

Adrenal Gland

The anatomic relationship of the adrenal gland to surrounding structures is the same as that described in the transperitoneal approach. However, the approach to the adrenal vein is quite different. Unlike in the transperitoneal approach, the left renal vein need not be dissected at all. Rather, the adrenal vein is seen just cranial to the pulsations of the left renal artery. Furthermore, it courses approximately 0.5–1 cm anterior and parallel to the horizon of the anterior psoas muscle (Figures 3.19 and 3.20).

The process of freeing the adrenal gland from its attachments is similar to that in the right retroperitoneal approach. Specifically, the gland is first freed of its cranial attachments to the peritoneum underlying the spleen, then of its anteromedial attachments to the peritoneum, and lastly of its cranial attachments from the superior surface of the bared kidney.

Caveats: When dissecting the posteromedial attachments of the adrenal gland, lateral traction (toward the surgeon) should be applied to the adrenal gland so that just the attachments connected to the adrenal gland are divided. This step further minimizes the chances of injury to the superior mesenteric artery.

2
Laparoscopic Anatomy of the Pelvis

Intra-Abdominal Anatomy of the Male Pelvic Region

A view of the anterior pelvic wall within the abdomen shows three cord-like peritoneal folds that appear to attach the bladder to the umbilicus: the median umbilical ligament (or median umbilical fold) and two medial umbilical ligaments (or medial umbilical folds). The median umbilical ligament extends from the dome of the bladder to the umbilicus and corresponds to the remnants of the fetal urachus. The medial umbilical ligaments arise from the pelvis as a continuation of the internal iliac artery and extend to the umbilicus. These are the obliterated segments of the fetal hypogastric arteries. More laterally, the lateral umbilical ligaments consist of peritoneal folds covering the epigastric vessels. Further laterally, the spermatic vessels can be visualized entering the deep inguinal ring (Figure 2.1).

Bladder

The dome of the bladder is the mobile portion of the bladder, and it stands out centrally. The anatomic relationships of the bladder change according to its level of fullness. Because a Foley catheter must be inserted into the bladder before the pneumoperitoneum is created, the bladder is initially empty and its limits are not clearly demarcated. As the bladder fills, its limits become more clearly delineated. Laterally, it expands toward the medial umbilical ligaments; anterior and superiorly, it expands toward the median umbilical ligament and the umbilicus, to which it is attached through the urachus.

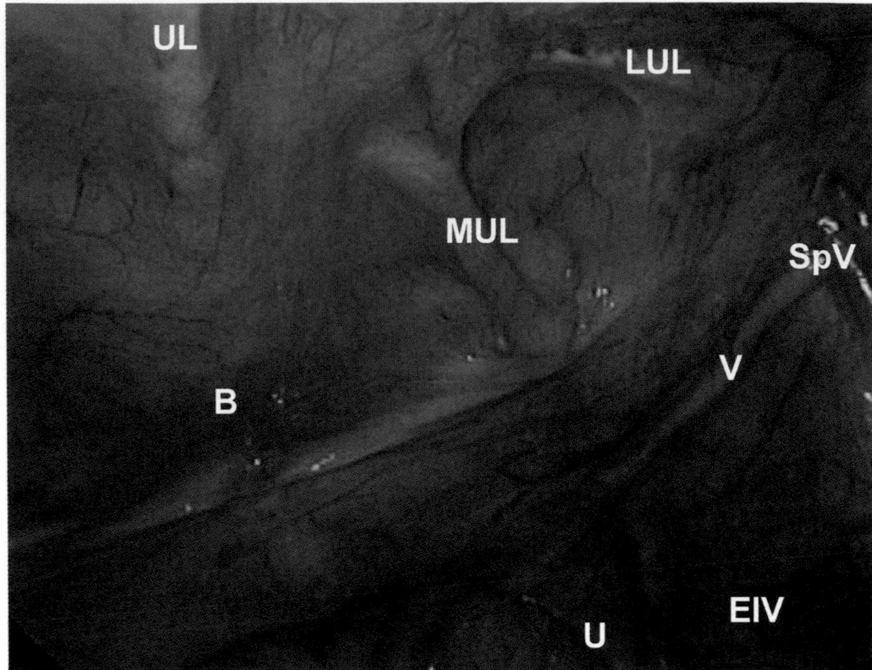

FIGURE 2.1. Umbilical ligaments (transperitoneal view of right hemipelvis). UL = median umbilical ligament, MUL = medial umbilical ligament, LUL = lateral umbilical ligament, B = bladder, V = vas deferens, SpV = spermatic vessels, EIV = external iliac vein, U = ureter

The median umbilical ligament (urachus) constitutes a fibromuscular cord, broad at its attachment to the bladder but narrowing as it ascends. It is a vascularized structure with few vessels that need to be controlled during dissection of the bladder. This fulguration can be avoided in case the urachus is spared. Laterally, the median umbilical ligament is separated from the medial umbilical ligament by the medial umbilical fossa, an anatomic landmark to access the space of Retzius.

It is important to emphasize the coalescence of the urachus and medial umbilical ligaments to the anterior parietal peritoneal wall during embryologic development to understand the planes that need to be incised during avascular access to the space of Retzius. Similar to the coalescence of the colonic gutters to the parietal peritoneal wall to form the fascias of Toldt, both the urachus and umbilical ligaments coalesce to the anterior parietal peritoneal wall; this is the plane that must be identified and developed to dissect the bladder off the anterior wall in a bloodless field (see LAPAROSCOPIC RADICAL PROSTATECTOMY, Chapter 9).

The pouch of Douglas (Figure 2.2) appears as a cul-de-sac between the bladder anteriorly and the rectum posteriorly. Its depth varies among patients, and it is used to make a posterior approach to the seminal vesicles. The exact location of the seminal vesicles cannot be readily visualized, but they are often found about 2 cm above the deepest part of the pouch of Douglas. The outline of the seminal vesicles and the distal portions of the vas deferens are occasionally visible in thin patients.

The visceral peritoneum and the underlying fat, which compose the anterior aspect of the pouch of Douglas that covers the bladder posteriorly, are rich in small vessels that should be fulgurated when incised to gain access to the seminal vesicles so that the surgical field is kept as bloodless as possible.

Medial Umbilical Ligaments

In the fetus, the hypogastric artery is twice as large as the external iliac artery, and it is the direct continuation of the common iliac artery. It ascends

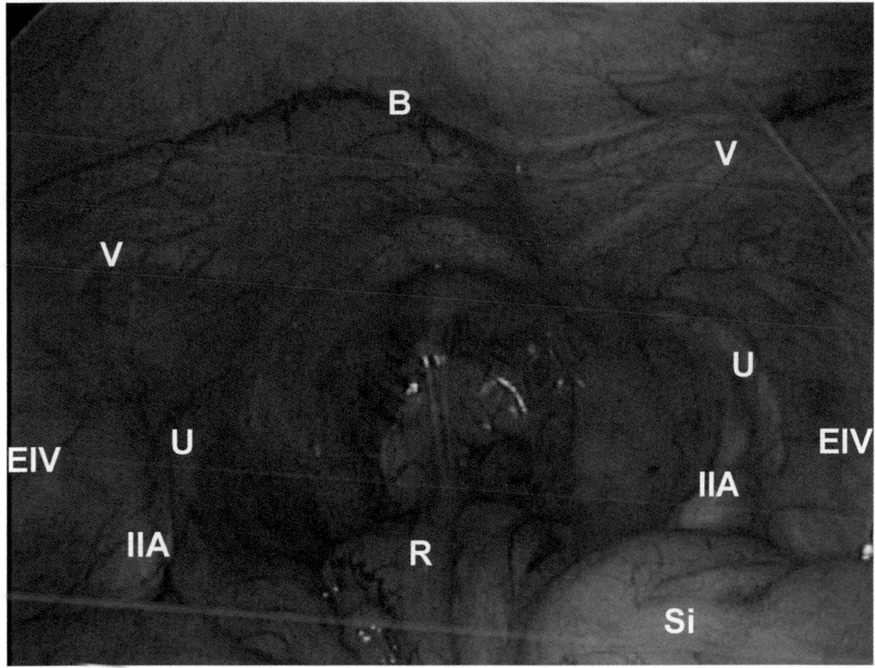

FIGURE 2.2. Pouch of Douglas. B = bladder, V = vas deferens, U = ureter, IIA = internal iliac artery, EIV = external iliac vein, R = rectum, Si = sigmoid colon

along the side of the bladder and runs upward on the back of the anterior abdominal wall to converge at the umbilicus with the hypogastric artery of the opposite side. Having passed through the umbilical opening, the two arteries, now termed umbilical, enter the umbilical cord, where they are coiled around the umbilical vein, and ultimately ramify in the placenta.

At birth, when the placental circulation ceases, only the pelvic portion of the artery remains patent and constitutes the hypogastric and the first part of the superior vesical artery in the adult; the remainder of the umbilical artery is converted into a solid fibrous cord, the medial umbilical ligament. This ligament is rarely vascularized and most often completely obliterated. The prominence of the medial umbilical ligaments varies depending on the amount of adipose tissue around it. The medial umbilical ligaments are particularly easy to see in laparoscopy and represent an important anatomic landmark for dissection not only of the pelvic lymph nodes but also of Retzius' space.

The ureter travels over the iliac vessels to run medial and deep to the medial umbilical ligament. Therefore, as long as the surgeon is able to visualize the umbilical ligament during pelvic lymph node dissection and dissect lateral to it, the ureter will not be at risk (see Chapter 7).

Laterally, the medial umbilical ligament is separated from the lateral umbilical ligament (the fold of peritoneum covering the inferior epigastric artery) by the medial umbilical fossa. This fossa is transversely divided into two portions by the vas deferens to form a quadrangle anteriorly and a triangle posteriorly. While the anterior quadrangle delimits an avascular access to Retzius' space, the posterior triangle is crucial to gain access to the obturator fossa for pelvic lymph node dissection. The vas deferens forms its base anteriorly, the external iliac vein laterally, and the medial umbilical ligament medially; the ureter can be visualized at the apex of the triangle (as it crosses over the iliac vessels) as well as deep on its medial aspect (Figure 2.3).

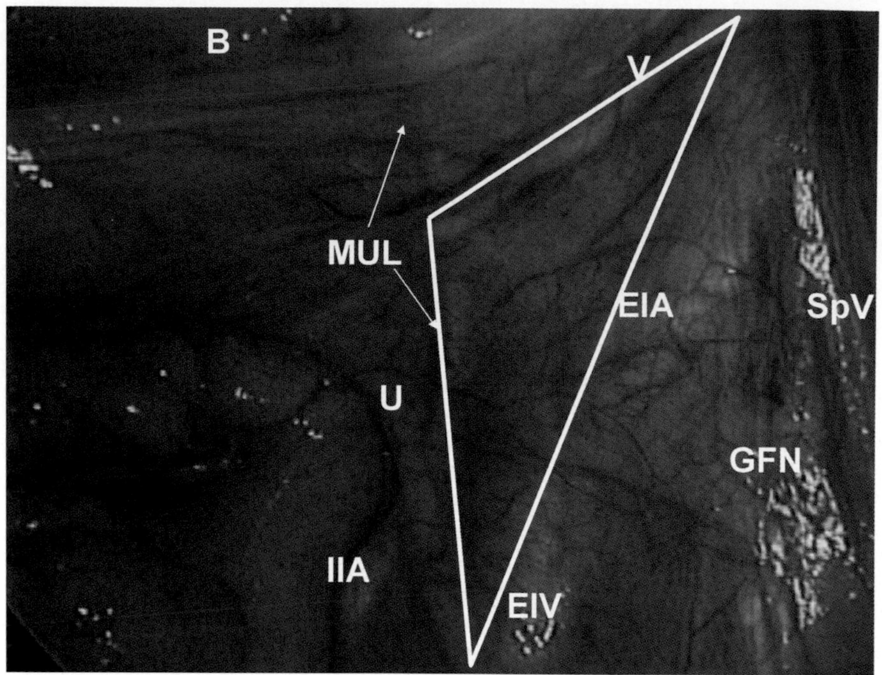

FIGURE 2.3. Base of vasculodeferential triangle composed of vas deferens (V) anteriorly, of medial umbilical ligament (MUL) medially, and of medial aspect of external iliac vein (EIV) laterally; triangle contains obturator lymph nodes along with obturator nerve and vessels (not visible). SpV = spermatic vessels, EIA = external iliac artery, GFN = genitofemoral nerve, B = bladder, U = ureter, IIA = internal iliac artery

Lateral Umbilical Ligaments

The inferior epigastric artery is a medial branch of the distal segment of the external iliac artery. It ascends along the medial margin of the deep inguinal ring, continues between the rectus abdominis muscle and the posterior lamina of its sheath, and then abuts on the anterior parietal peritoneum to create the lateral umbilical ligament. This ligament is the least pronounced of the three aforementioned peritoneal folds, and it is not always readily visualized. However, knowledge of its location is important to avoid injury to these vessels during either insertion of the lateral trocars or dissection of the space of Retzius.

Spermatic Cords

The spermatic cord is formed by the convergence of the lymphovascular packet draining the testes, the vas deferens, the corresponding nerves (the genital branch of the genitofemoral nerve and the ilioinguinal and sympathetic spermatic plexus), and the gonadal vessels. The gonadal artery runs over the iliopsoas muscle and joins the vas deferens before entering the deep inguinal ring. The gonadal veins ascend on the psoas major, behind the peritoneum, lying on each side of the gonadal artery. They unite to form a single vein, which opens on the right side at an acute angle into the inferior vena cava, and on the left side at a right angle into the left renal vein.

The vas deferens is rarely visible at the posterolateral aspect of the prostate but becomes more visible as its course becomes more superficial laterally as it crosses over the external iliac vessels.

Again, the vas deferens and the medial umbilical ligament are major landmarks for pelvic lymph node dissection: the vertical incision of the parietal peritoneum lateral to the medial umbilical ligament and posterior to the vas deferens provides the initial access to the obturator fossa. The external iliac vein can be immediately identified laterally, with the external iliac artery located further anterolaterally.

Iliac Vessels

The external iliac artery is easily recognized pulsating below the overlying parietal peritoneum fold at the level where the vas deferens joins the gonadal vessels.

Lateral to the external iliac artery is the genitofemoral nerve, which can eventually be used for nerve grafting after resection of the prostatic neurovascular bundle. The genitofemoral nerve descends on the surface of the psoas major, under cover of the peritoneum, and divides into the external spermatic and lumboinguinal nerves. The external spermatic nerve (the genital branch of the genitofemoral nerve) descends behind the spermatic cord to the scrotum, supplies the cremaster muscle, and provides a few filaments to the skin of the scrotum. The lumboinguinal nerve (the femoral branch of the genitofemoral), which descends superficial and lateral to the femoral artery, pierces the anterior layer of the sheath of the vessels and the fascia lata. It supplies the skin of the anterior surface of the upper part of the thigh.

The external iliac vein is medial and posterior to the external iliac artery. It can be masked by an aneurysmal or tortuous iliac artery. Furthermore, the pressure of the pneumoperitoneum compressing the vein can sometimes obscure its visualization. In this situation, delineation of the vein may be improved by decreasing the intra-abdominal pressure.

Longitudinal incision of the peritoneum lying over the medial umbilical ligament posterior to the vas deferens exposes the external iliac vein. Its medial aspect can be easily and safely dissected, except for its most distal segment where one or two veins branching medially can be identified. The first one is the accessory obturator vein, which comes off the obturator foramen to drain into the external iliac vein just posterior to Cloquet's node. The second is the venous component of the corona mortis, which is an anastomotic artery and vein between the epigastric and the obturator vessels. Proximally, the internal iliac or hypogastric vein, which composes the superior limit of the pelvic lymph node dissection, is identified going posteriorly. Dissection at the confluence of the internal and external iliac veins allows access first to the obturator nerve and, more posteriorly, to the superior vesical artery and superior gluteal vessels. The external iliac vessels are located more anteriorly on the right side than on the left.

The obturator nerve is located posterior and medial to the external iliac vein. It appears as a white, shining, striated, usually flattened cord that enters the obturator fossa distally. Proximally, it is located at the convergence of the internal and external iliac veins. The obturator artery, a primary or secondary branch of the internal or even external iliac artery, usually runs posterior to the obturator nerve, and the obturator vein is commonly located further posteriorly. Anatomic variations of the pelvic vessels are common, and careful dissection is always required to avoid their inadvertent injury.

The limits of the pelvic lymph node dissection are formed by the external iliac vein laterally, the medial umbilical ligament medially, the pelvic floor and the anterior surface of the hypogastric artery posteriorly, Cooper's ligament distally, and the bifurcation of the iliac vein proximally. In other words, the lymph nodes around both the obturator artery and external iliac vein are removed as well as those lying on the anterior aspect of the hypogastric artery (see Chapter 7).

Ureters

The ureters can be easily identified in two locations as soon as the pelvis is entered. The clearest one is where they cross over the common iliac vessels to then form the posteromedial limit of the pelvic lymph node dissection. Identification of the left ureter can be difficult when the sigmoid colon is adhered to the parietal peritoneum. In rare cases, depending on the patient's distribution of adipose tissue, the ureters can also be seen through the transparent lateral walls of the pouch of Douglas as they go below the vas deferens.

For this reason, the initial transverse incision on the anterior aspect of the pouch of Douglas to gain access to the seminal vesicles posteriorly should be no longer than 2 cm laterally to avoid any damage to the ureters as they pass below the vas deferens. In theory, the ureters should not be seen at this level; if they can be visualized, the incision has been continued too far laterally.

Seminal Vesicular Complex

The seminal vesicular complex is composed of the distal portion of the two vas deferens prolonged by the ampullae, and the two seminal vesicles. The entire complex is rarely visible through the visceral

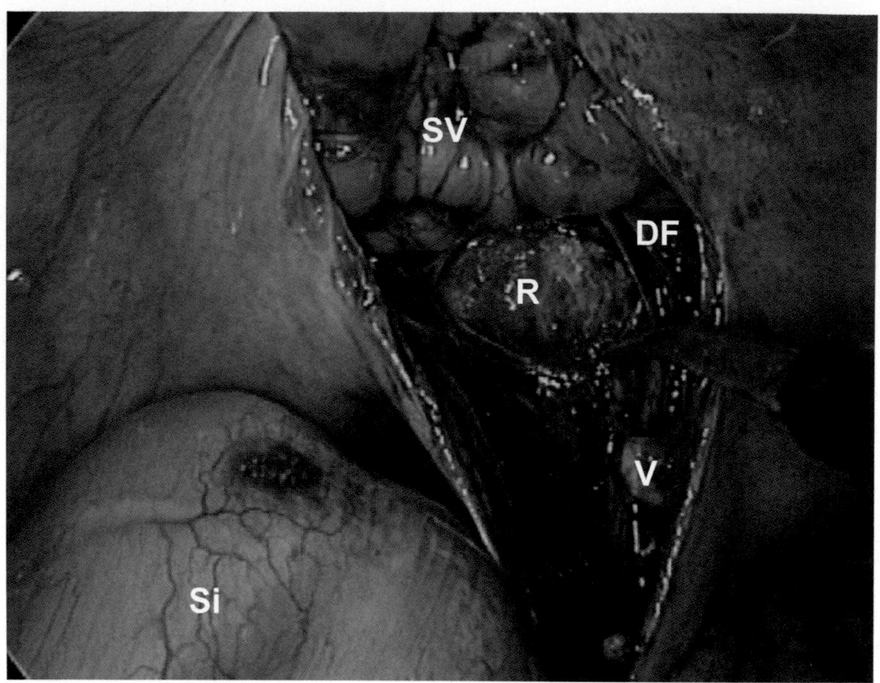

FIGURE 2.4. Transperitoneal view of Denonvilliers' fascia (DF) after its opening through incision of anterior peritoneal fold of pouch of Douglas; seminal vesicles (SV) and vas deferens (V) pulled anteriorly; anterior of rectum (R) covered by fatty layer. Si = sigmoid colon

peritoneal fold of the anterior aspect of the pouch of Douglas. However, depending on the size of the seminal vesicles and the amount of intra-abdominal fat, the seminal vesicular complex can be identified, which facilitates initial dissection of the structures. Transverse incision of the peritoneal fold about 2 cm above the base of the recess allows access to a thin layer of fibrous tissue covering the seminal vesicles (Figure 2.4). Transverse incision of this fascia exposes the vas deferens. Again, hemostasis is crucial because this peritoneal layer is lined with multiple small vessels. The deferential artery runs lateral to each vas (between the vas deferens and the seminal vesicles) and, more anteriorly, the seminal vesicles lie inferior and lateral to the vas deferens.

The anterior aspect (the one in contact with the prostate) and the tip of the seminal vesicles are highly vascularized, in contrast to the posterior face (the one contacting Denonvilliers' fascia), which is relatively hypovascular. Meticulous hemostasis of these vesicular vessels is crucial, because they can be a source of bleeding that could eventually require another surgery.

The lateral aspect and the tip of the seminal vesicles are close to the inferior hypogastric plexus (also known as the pelvic plexus), which innervates the pelvis. The inferior hypogastric plexus measures about 40 mm high, 10 mm wide, and 3 mm thick, and it is molded to the convolutions of the seminal vesicles. The inferior hypogastric plexus receives afferent fibers from the superior hypogastric plexus—or preaortic plexus (sympathetic fibers arising from the thoracic region)—and from the pelvic splanchnic nerves—or erector nerves (parasympathetic preganglionic fibers arising from the sacral plexus S2 to S4). The cavernous nerves emerge at the anteroinferior border of the inferior hypogastric plexus.

The close anatomic relationship between the inferior hypogastric plexus—which should not be seen during the surgery—and the seminal vesicle, especially at its tip, is the basis for a meticulous seminal vesicle dissection.

The seminal vesicle receives most of its arterial supply from the deferential artery, a characteristically tortuous branch of the vesiculodeferential artery, which invariably appears running in close relationship to the vas deferens and is identified immediately after sectioning the vas deferens when they are approached posteriorly, that is, through the pouch of Douglas.

Anterior traction on the vas deferens and seminal vesicles exposes Denonvilliers' fascia lying posterior to the seminal vesicular complex. This prostatorectal fascia appears as vertically striated tissue covering the seminal vesicular complex posteriorly, and its dissection leads to the prerectal space, which is filled with variable amounts of adipose tissue.

Dissection of the posterior bladder neck exposes the outer longitudinal muscle fibers of the bladder inserting into the base of the prostate, covering anteriorly the seminal vesicular complex. These fibers are covered by a layer of fibroadipose tissue that contains arteries and nerves and that is a continuation of the adventitia of the bladder. This double layer of tissue (smooth muscle of the outer longitudinal muscle fibers of the bladder and fibroadipose tissue), often misinterpreted as "anterior Denonvilliers' fascia," must be incised to gain access to the vas deferens and the seminal vesicles. This structure is clearly recognized by the longitudinal disposition of the muscle fibers (Figure 2.5).

Rectum and Sigmoid Colon

Only the superior half of the rectum is visible during laparoscopy of the pelvis. Having the patient in the Trendelenburg position allows for superior mobilization of the sigmoid colon by gravity and for inspection of the pouch of Douglas. Because the sigmoid colon coalesces with the parietal peritoneum, dissection is occasionally required to adequately mobilize the sigmoid colon out of the pouch of Douglas before the seminal vesicles can be dissected. The left pelvic lymph node dissection also requires detachment of the sigmoid colon from the peritoneal wall. This dissection should be done with care because the ureter, the iliac artery, or even the gonadal vessels can be found immediately underneath the sigmoid colon.

Retropublic Space

The retropubic space can be approached laparoscopically either transperitoneally or preperitoneally.

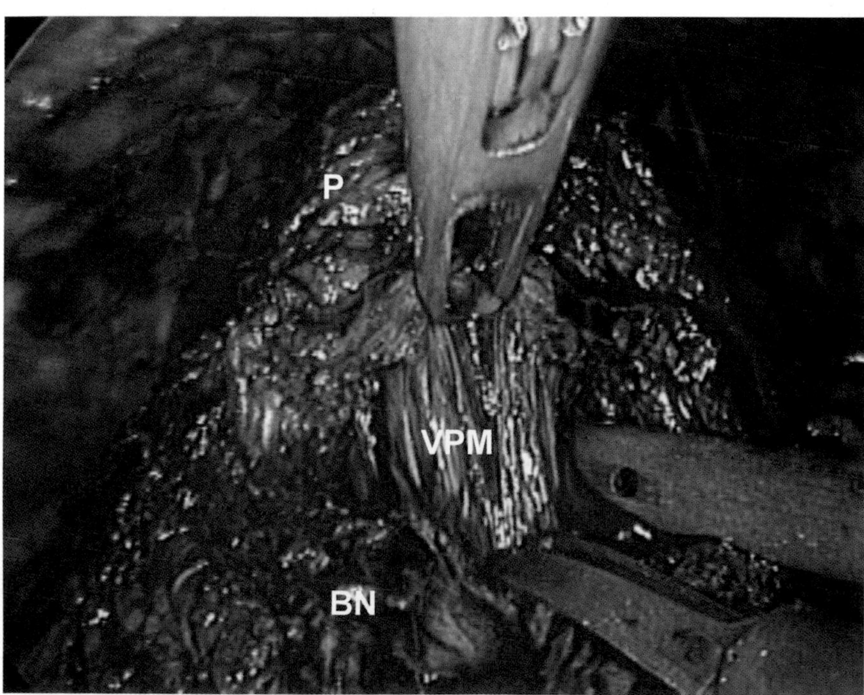

FIGURE 2.5. Longitudinally disposed muscle fibers corresponding to longitudinal fascia of detrusor muscle (not to be confused with anterior layer of Denonvilliers' fascia). BN = bladder neck, VPM = vesicoprostatic muscle, P = prostate

In the sagittal plane, the retropubic space forms a triangle, limited anteriorly by the fascia transversalis and the anterior parietal peritoneum covering the posterior surface of the anterior abdominal wall, inferiorly by the pubis, and posteriorly by the bladder through the umbilicoprevesical fascia and the endopelvic fascia. The retropubic space is lined laterally by the internal obturator muscles.

Pubis

The superior ramus of the pubic bone is covered by Cooper's ligament, a strong fibrous band that extends laterally from the insertion of the inguinal ligament into the pubic tubercle along the pectineal line, to which it is attached. It is strengthened by the pectineal fascia and by a lateral expansion from the lower attachment of the linea alba. Cooper's ligament is an important landmark to identify the correct plane during the dissection of the space of Retzius.

Osteophytes may be encountered after developing the space of Retzius. However, unlike in open surgery, osteophytes covering the pubic symphysis seldom obscure visualization.

Obturator Muscles

On each side of the pelvis, the obturator muscle is "tented" between the ischial spine and the inferior border of the pubic ramus and is supported inferiorly by the tendinous arch of the levator ani muscle. The obturator muscle covers the obturator foramen and leaves passage to the obturator pedicle through the obturator canal. The muscle constitutes the lateral limit of the pelvic lymph node dissection.

Bladder

Gaining access to the prostate does not require mobilization of the entire bladder. Access can be achieved simply by opening Retzius' space, which is filled with a layer of lax tissue and varying amounts of fat. The anterior bladder wall can be easily dissected off the pubic bone and the transversalis fascia, which covers the posterior aspect of the rectus muscle aponeurosis.

Laterally, the bladder is attached to the pelvic cavity via the vesical ligament which carries, from top to bottom, the obliterated umbilical artery, the superior vesical artery and veins, the distal portion of the ureter, and inferiorly the inferior vesical artery and veins. The origin of both the inferior vesical and prostatic arteries is variable. However, the presence of a branch that joins the cavernous nerves to form the so-called "neurovascular bundle" is relatively constant. This branch can provide vital vascularization to both the nerves and the sphincteric complex, the preservation of which may substantially contribute to retaining potency and continence. After the prostate has been removed, the preservation of the cavernous arteries can be easily evaluated with the aid of a Doppler probe. Preservation of the cavernous arteries can be used as a surrogate for preservation of the cavernous nerves.

Endopelvic Fascia

The endopelvic fascia is the inferior limit of the space of Retzius. It stretches from one tendinous arch of the levator ani muscle to the other, covering the anterior aspect of the prostate.

Laterally, the endopelvic fascia forms two recesses (or sulci) between the prostate medially and the muscles of the pelvic wall laterally. These recesses are incised to approach the lateral aspects of the prostate. The endopelvic fascia is particularly weak toward the base of the prostate, where it is thinner than its anterior aspect, which is reinforced by the puboprostatic ligaments.

As stated earlier, an accessory pudendal artery can sometimes be identified on the superior surface of the endopelvic fascia, and it should be preserved because it may represent the single major source of blood supply to the corpus cavernosum.

The incision of the endopelvic fascia should start proximally because of the paucity of blood vessels near the base of the gland. This incision uncovers the medial aspect of the levator ani muscle, which is covered by the levator ani fascia (also called lateral pelvic fascia) below the tendinous arch. Although it is possible to dissect medial to the levator ani fascia, ie, between itself and the prostatic fascia, sometimes the dissection is done more laterally. In this case, the levator ani fascia is left attached to the prostatic fascia, and the levator ani fibers become exposed. Inferiorly, the prostatic fascia fuses with Denonvilliers' fascia to delimit the course of the branches of the cavernous nerve and the neurovascular bundle.

More anteriorly, posterior to the lateral oblique extension of the puboprostatic ligament, vessels arising through fibers of the levator ani muscle toward the superolateral aspect of the prostatic apex may be identified. In approximately 15% of patients, an accessory pudendal artery can be identified coming through the fibers of the levator ani muscle and running to the anterolateral aspect of the prostatic apex where it turns toward the penis and runs parallel to the vascular complex after giving one or two branches to the apex (apical accessory pudendal artery). This main trunk may also supply the corpus cavernosum and should be preserved.

Anteriorly, the puboprostatic ligament combines with the endopelvic fascia attached to the inferior border of the inferior pubic ramus, where it merges with the extension of the falciform process of the sacrotuberous ligament (a strong supporting ligament that joins the sacrum to the ischial tuberosity and forms the inferior border of the lesser sciatic foramen). On each side, the puboprostatic ligament is either single and vertical, or multiple often with a lateral oblique extension (Figure 2.6). In a sagittal plane, the most medial ligament is not a cord tethered between the pubis and the prostatic apex, but more a fold that is continuous with the transverse perineal ligament (arcuate pubic ligament).

Histologically, the puboprostatic ligaments are extensions of the detrusor muscle (detrusor apron) that partially cover the anterior surface of the prostate; hence the name "pubovesical ligaments" would be more correct anatomically. For that reason, completely preserving these ligaments (in reference to so-called puboprostatic ligament-sparing techniques) is anatomically impossible because without incising them, at least partially, there is no way of obtaining access to the deep vascular complex and the urethra.

In between the pubic attachments of the puboprostatic ligaments emerges one (or occasionally more) superficial dorsal vein separated from the deep vascular complex by a lax plane that can be easily developed. Frequently, this vein runs within the fat covering the anterior layer of the endopelvic fascia and gives one or more branches at the level of the vesicoprostatic junction, where it enters the detrusor muscle. In some patients, this vein bifurcates or trifurcates immediately after it enters the

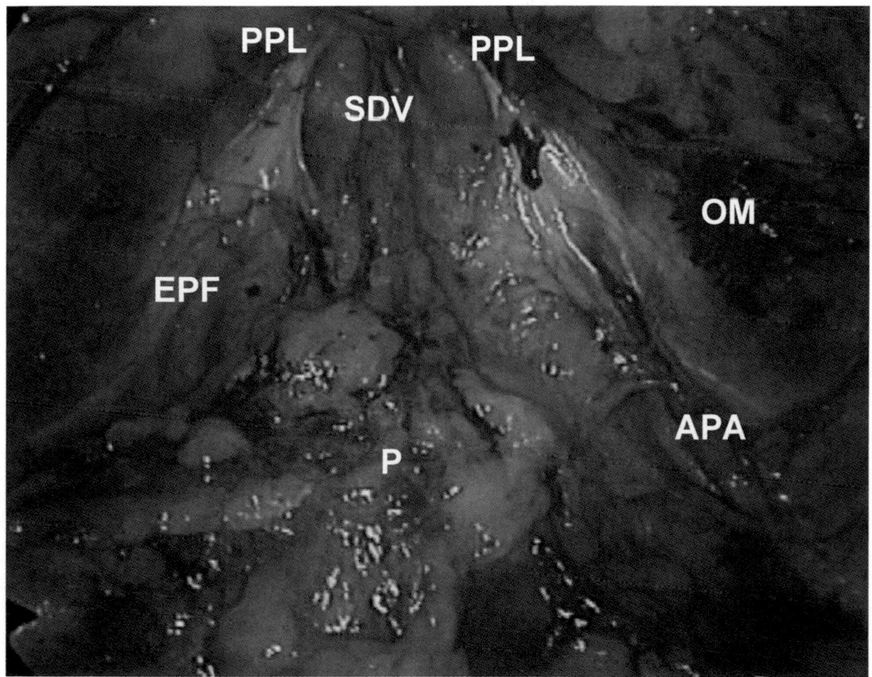

FIGURE 2.6. Retropubic space showing fat covering anterior aspect of endopelvic fascia (EPF); lateral accessory pudendal artery (APA) on right side, crossing below right sulcus of endopelvic fascia. PPL = puboprostatic ligaments, SDV = superficial dorsal vein, OM = obturator muscle; P = prostate

pelvis into branches that run on the internal layer of the rectus abdominis or obturator muscles.

The puboprostatic ligaments are not vascularized and can be cut safely. Laterally, the puboprostatic ligament fuses with the extension of the parietal fascia of the levator ani muscle and with the visceral prostatic fascia into a relatively thick "sphincteric" fascia that covers the lateral aspect of the deep vascular complex. More posteriorly, this sphincteric fascia covers the ischioprostatic ligaments—also known as Müller's ligaments—that anchor the rhabdomyosphincter with the sphincteric urethra to the bony structures.

Santorini's Plexus

Santorini's plexus is composed of the superficial dorsal vein (described above) and the so-called "deep vascular complex" (Figure 2.7). Because this complex is composed of large veins draining the penis, and one or two arteries, the name "deep vascular complex" is more appropriate than "deep venous complex."

These arteries are not terminal branches; when transected, bleeding from the distal end is pulsatile. It is assumed that their transection does not affect continence or erectile function given that they are retrograde branches of the internal pudendal arteries that supply the anterior surface of the prostate and bladder.

Superiorly, the Santorini's plexus branches into a network of veins and arteries on the anterior aspect of the prostate. Some of the veins penetrate the prostatic apron and drain into the prostatic pedicular veins; others drain directly into the pudendal veins along the neurovascular bundles.

Prostatic Fascia and Prostatic Pedicles

Prostatic Fascia

The visceral prostatic fascia covers the external surface of the prostate. On the posterolateral surface of the prostate, the prostatic fascia is continuous with Denonvilliers' fascia, and it can be dissected off the prostatic capsule delineating the medial surface of the neurovascular bundle. This plane of dissection between the prostatic capsule and the prostatic fascia leaves the neurovascular bundle

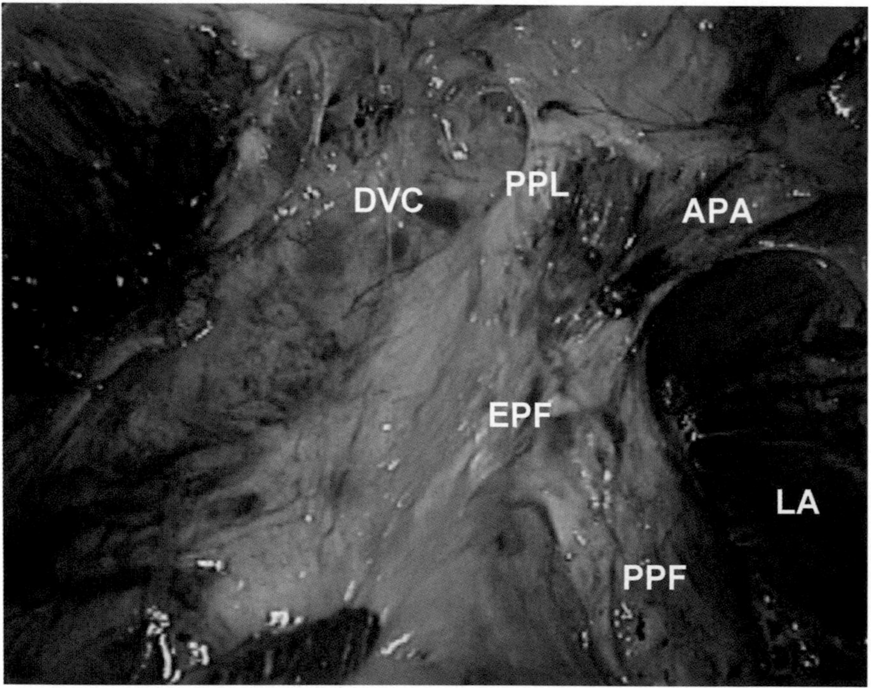

FIGURE 2.7. Apex of prostate; Santorini's plexus has been ligated and divided. DVC = deep vascular complex, PPL = puboprostatic ligament, APA = accessory pudendal artery, EPF = endopelvic fascia, PPF = periprostatic fascia, LA = levator ani muscle

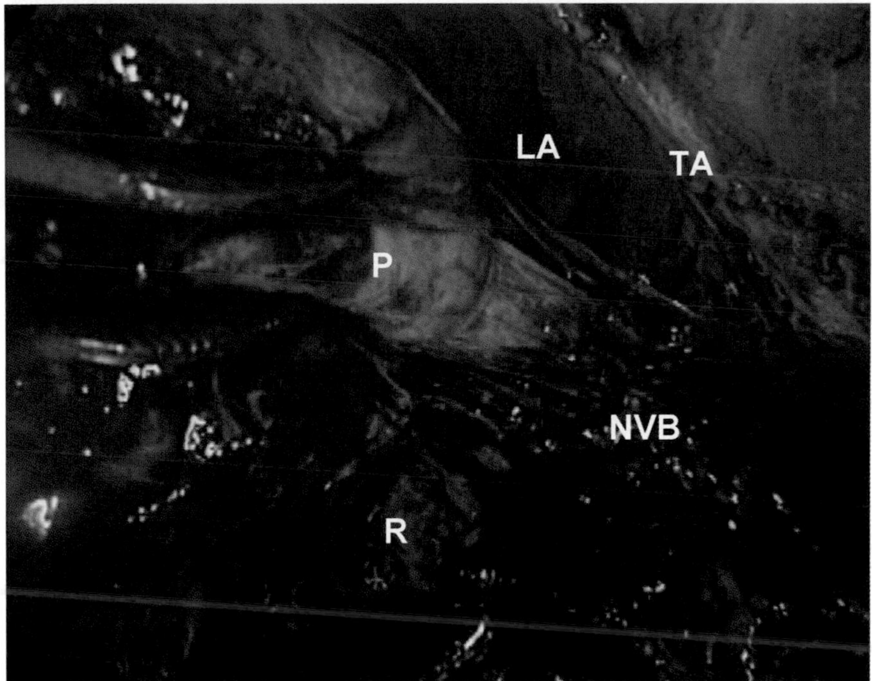

FIGURE 2.8. Right neurovascular bundle (NVB) covered by its fascia; fusion of prostatic fascia and Denonvilliers' fascia. P = prostate, LA = levator ani muscle, TA = tendinous arch of levator ani muscle, R = rectum

totally intact, surrounded by this fascia. In this situation, the cavernous nerves, the vessels of the neurovascular bundle, and the fatty tissue in which they are embedded are not directly seen. This dissection can be considered "intrafascial" neurovascular bundle dissection (Figure 2.8) versus "interfascial" dissection, in which dissection is performed between the prostatic fascia and Denonvilliers' fascia with variable degrees of penetration into the neurovascular bundle itself. In this case, the elements of the neurovascular bundle are exposed, and the prostatic fascia fusing with Denonvilliers' fascia stays on the prostate side rather than covering the internal aspect of the neurovascular bundle. In this situation, the structures of the neurovascular bundle are at risk of damage during their dissection. The term "extrafascial" dissection implies that the dissection is performed lateral to the entire neurovascular bundle. In this case, the neurovascular bundle is completely or almost completely resected (Figure 2.9).

Denonvilliers' Fascia

Denonvilliers' fascia is also known as the "posterior prostatorectal fascia," "septum rectovesicale," or "prostatoseminal vesicular fascia." Denonvilliers' fascia is posterior to the prostate and anterior to the rectum. Inferiorly, Denonvilliers' fascia merges with the expansions of the rectourethralis muscle, posterior to the sphincteric membranous urethra. Laterally, it merges with the lateral fold of the prostatic fascia, forming the superior-medial and inferior-medial borders of the neurovascular bundle.

Denonvilliers' fascia is more adherent to the prostate than to the rectum, particularly on its superior aspect where it is separated from the rectum by a layer of fatty tissue (the mesorectum); distally Denonvilliers' fascia becomes much more adherent to the rectal wall. Because Denonvilliers' fascia contains nerves that enter the prostate gland and can be involved in invasive cancer, it should be routinely removed along with the radical prostatectomy specimen.

A common misunderstanding indicates that the "anterior layer of Denonvilliers' fascia" is a layer of tissue that needs to be incised to access and dissect both the vas deferens and seminal vesicles from the posterior bladder neck. However, anatomic descriptions do not support the presence

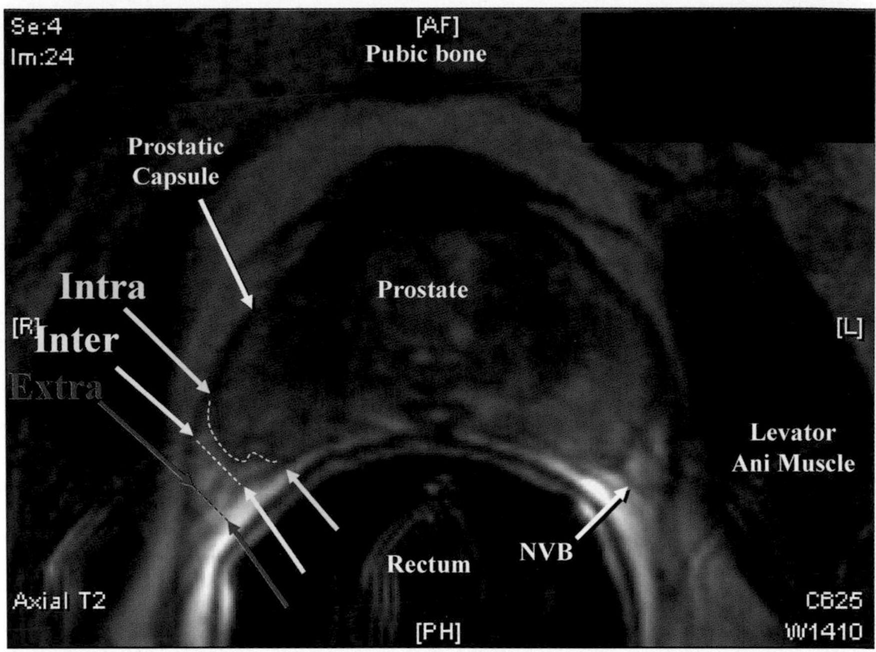

FIGURE 2.9. Different planes of neurovascular bundle (NVB) dissection as depicted on axial T2 weighed section of prostate on endorectal coil magnetic resonance imaging. Intra = intrafascia, Inter = interfascial, Extra = extrafascial planes of dissection

of Denonvilliers' fascia anterior to the seminal vesicles. These longitudinally oriented fibers, which are identified after the posterior bladder neck has been incised, are not an "anterior layer of Denonvilliers' fascia"; rather, they are the longitudinal fascicle of the detrusor muscle. These muscle fibers are covered externally by a layer of fibroadipose tissue that is continuous with the adventitia of the bladder (Figure 2.5).

Rectourethralis Muscle

The Y-shaped rectourethralis muscle is not frequently encountered in laparoscopy because it arises within the substance of the rectal wall deep to the outer longitudinal smooth muscle and inserts into the central tendon of the peritoneum. It is accepted that Denonvilliers' fascia inserts distally on the rectourethralis muscle, with which it merges.

Prostatic Neurovascular Plexus

The prostatic neurovascular plexus contains veins, arteries, and autonomic nerves. Despite the spray-like distribution of the autonomic nerve fibers emerging from the inferior hypogastric plexus (pelvic plexus) on the dorsolateral aspect of the prostate, the bulk of the cavernous nerves and vessels is limited by the fascia of the levator ani muscle laterally, Denonvilliers' fascia posteromedially, and the prostatic fascia anteromedially.

Cavernous Nerves: The cavernous nerves, which are both sympathetic and parasympathetic autonomic nerves, arise from the inferior hypogastric plexus. These nerves appear like a network that distributes to the prostate and to the corpus cavernosum. The cavernous nerves join the prostatic artery at the level of the pedicle. The branches of the nerve network then follow the posterolateral aspect of the prostate toward the apex, accompanied by veins and branches of the prostatic pedicular artery. Apically, the nerves run more posteromedially to the prostate. Along their course, small branches of the cavernous nerves penetrate the prostatic capsule. However, these branching intracapsular nerves are rarely seen on the lateral aspect of the prostate and become more evident either at the base or apex of the prostate.

Arteries: The arteries are well visualized during laparoscopic dissection and are important landmarks for initiating the "intrafascial" neurovascular dissection (Figure 2.10). At the level of the arborescence

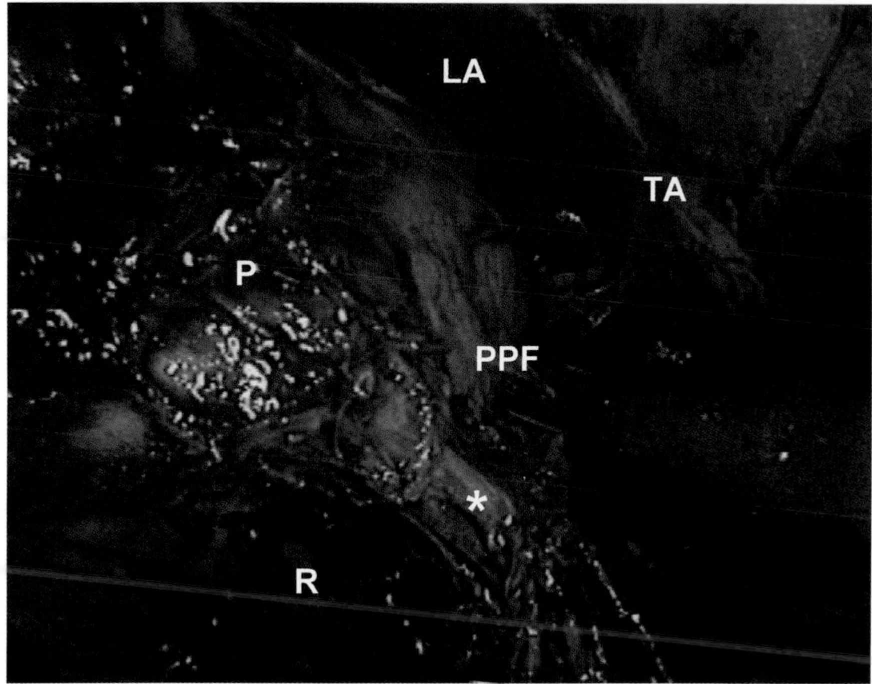

FIGURE 2.10. Right prostatic pedicle. * = main prostatic pedicular artery with its vein, PPF = periprostatic fascia, LA = levator ani muscle, TA = tendinous arch of levator ani muscle, P = prostate, R = rectum

of the prostatic arteries into prostatic, vesicular, and deferential arteries, at least one branch runs anterior to the bulk of the cavernous nerves on the posterolateral aspect of the prostate.

Once within the neurovascular bundle, the artery divides into an arterial network. Rarely, one of these arteries crosses the medial prostatic fascia to enter the prostatic capsule at the mid portion of the gland. More often, the arteries run all along the prostate and give a retrograde branch only to the apex.

Veins: The veins follow the course of the artery, but not infrequently, a large vein coming from the deep vascular complex runs on the anterior tip of the crescent-shaped neurovascular bundle. This vein can be used as a landmark for neurovascular bundle preservation.

Accessory Pudendal Arteries

Accessory pudendal arteries are defined as any artery located within the periprostatic region that run parallel to the dorsal vascular complex and extend caudally toward the anterior perineum to contribute to the blood supply (in different degrees) of the corpus cavernosum. They can be identified in approximately 30% of patients undergoing laparoscopic radical prostatectomy.

Two distinct varieties of accessory pudendal arteries can be identified: those coursing along the lateral aspect of the prostate, termed *lateral* accessory pudendal arteries, and those running near the apical region of the prostate, termed *apical* accessory pudendal arteries.

Lateral accessory pudendal arteries are found in three possible locations: in intimate contact with the anterolateral prostatic surface, in intimate contact with the endopelvic fascia, or in intimate contact with the posterior surface of the pubic bone (termed pubic lateral accessory pudendal arteries) (Figure 2.11).

Apical accessory pudendal arteries are identified inferior and lateral to the pubovesical ligaments (Figure 2.12). They emerge through the levator ani muscle fibers and tangentially approach the prostatic apex. Their course, unlike that of the lateral accessory pudendal arteries, is not along the lateral aspect of the prostate but directly to the prostatic apex. Apical accessory pudendal arteries are usually exposed after both the endopelvic fascia and the levator ani fascia are incised at the level of the apex.

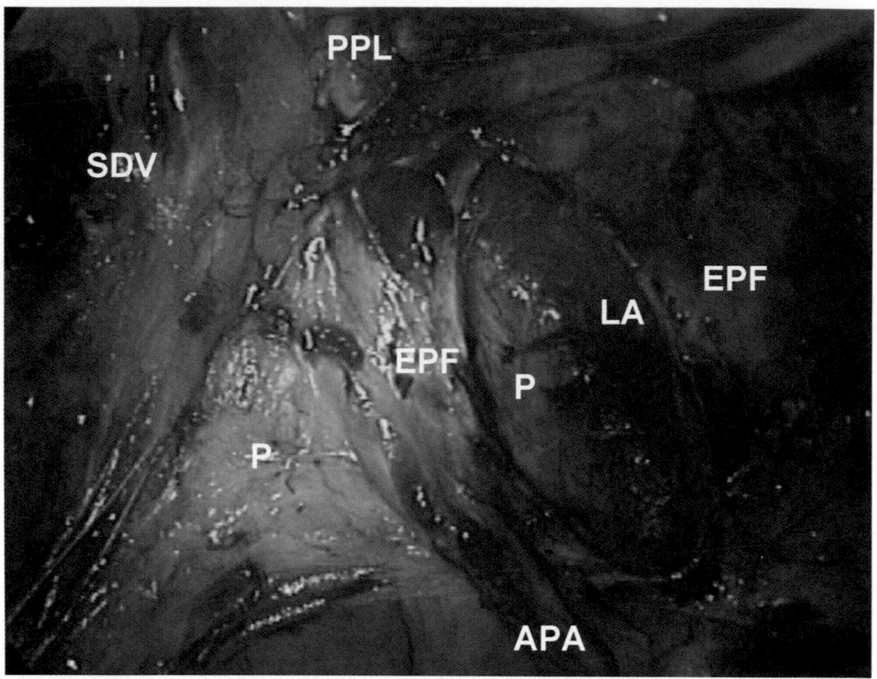

FIGURE 2.11. Fascial lateral accessory pudendal artery (APA) runs on right anterior aspect of endopelvic fascia (EPF) before piercing fascia and running along anterolateral aspect of prostate (P). LA = levator ani muscle, PPL = puboprostatic ligament, SDV = superficial dorsal vein

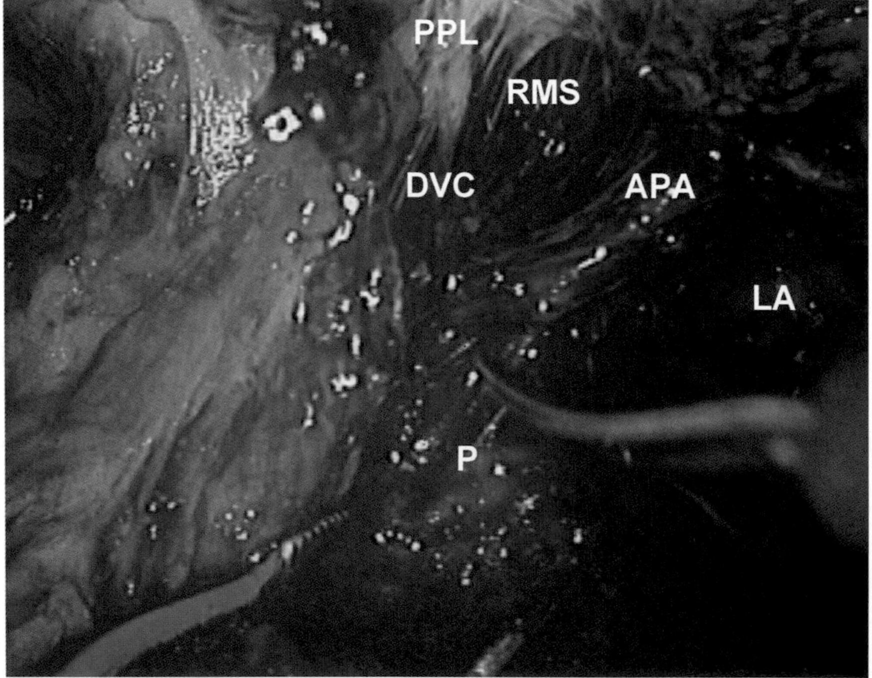

FIGURE 2.12. Apical accessory pudendal artery (APA) identified inferior and lateral to puboprostatic ligaments (PPL), emerging through levator ani muscle (LA) fibers and tangentially approaching prostatic apex, lateral to deep vascular complex (DVC). P = prostate, RMS = rhabdomyosphincter

As the lateral or apical accessory pudendal arteries extend toward the deep vascular complex, a collateral branch to the prostatic apex can be identified in approximately 50% of the patients. Lateral and/or apical accessory pudendal arteries continue along the lateral aspect of the veins of the deep vascular complex underneath the pubic arch, toward the anterior perineum.

Both lateral and apical accessory pudendal arteries are unilateral in approximately 80% of patients with accessory pudendal arteries and bilateral in 20%. Apical accessory pudendal arteries tend to be smaller in diameter and are more frequently identified on the left side, which make their preservation more difficult. A very small number of patients (1%) have a combination of lateral and apical accessory pudendal arteries.

Identification and preservation of accessory pudendal arteries might play a role in recovery of erectile function in patients undergoing nerve-sparing prostatectomy. However, the impact of their preservation on both recovery of erectile function and urinary continence after prostatectomy has yet to be determined.

Sphincteric Complex

Urethra

An avascular plane exists between the deep vascular complex and the anterior surface of the urethra. This plane must be recognized intraoperatively after incising the deep vascular complex, because it is the only way to identify the contour of the prostatic apex and therefore avoid an apical positive surgical margin.

After sectioning the urethra, the urethral stump is usually retracted to some degree.

Rhabdomyosphincter

The detrusor, trigone, and urethral sphincter muscles all contribute to urinary continence. The external urethral sphincter covers the ventral surface of the prostate as a crescent-shaped structure above the veru montanum, assumes a horseshoe shape below the veru montanum, and then becomes more crescent-shaped again along the proximal bulbar urethra. The levator ani muscles form an open circle around the external sphincter (ie, they are not completely closed at the ventral aspect). The smooth and striated muscle components of the urethral sphincteric complex cannot be distinguished from one another or separated.

The length of the sphincteric urethra (as measured by magnetic resonance imaging) is variable, ranging from 6 to 24 mm (average 14 mm) and seems to be directly related to recovery of urinary continence.

Innervation of the Rhabdomyosphincter: The innervation of the so-called "rhabdomyosphincter" is supported mainly by fibers coming from S2-S4 roots, traveling via the pudendal nerve. These nerves are not seen during the laparoscopic approach to the pelvis, because they run posterolateral to the rectum and then inferior to the levator ani muscle. The main trunk accompanies the internal pudendal vessels upward and forward along the lateral wall of the ischiorectal fossa (being contained in a sheath of the obturator fascia termed Alcock's canal) and, after having given off the inferior hemorrhoidal nerve, divides into two terminal branches, viz, the perineal nerve and the dorsal nerve of the penis. The perineal nerve is located below the internal pudendal artery. It accompanies the perineal artery and divides into posterior scrotal and muscular branches. The muscular branches are distributed to the superficial transverse perineal, bulbocavernosus, ischiocavernous, and urethral sphincter muscles. Some extrapudendal nerves can also be found (although not consistently) inside the pelvis and may be damaged during surgery. Rhabdomyosphincteric innervation by branches arising from the pelvic plexus (S4 root) has also been described (as a branch of the pelvic splanchnic nerve), but these branches are also posterolateral to the rectum and not visible during pelvic dissection.

Intra-Abdominal Anatomy of the Female Pelvic Region

Overview and Compartments

The female pelvis is more nearly circular in contour than the male pelvis. The obvious laparoscopic differences between the male and female pelvis include the presence of the internal genitalia and the adnexal structures interposed between the bladder and rectum. The peritoneum covers these pelvic organs, creating additional folds and ligaments that serve as visual landmarks (Figure 2.13).

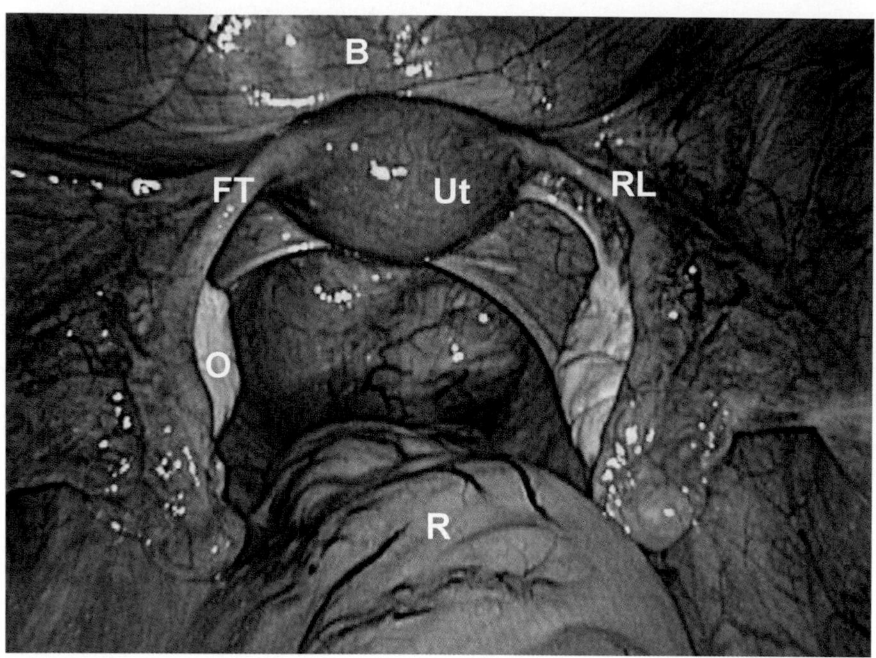

FIGURE 2.13. Normal female pelvic anatomy. B = bladder, FT = fallopian tube, O = ovary, R = rectum, RL = round ligament, Ut = uterus

Transperitoneal access of the female pelvic cavity allows visualization of three compartments in the midline: the anterior, the middle, and the posterior compartments. The anterior compartment is occupied by the bladder and urethra. It is limited by the pubic symphysis anteriorly and the vesicouterine fold posteriorly. The vesicouterine fold separates the anterior from the middle compartment.

The middle compartment is occupied by the vagina, cervix, and uterus medially, and by the round ligaments, fallopian tubes, and ovaries more laterally. The middle compartment is separated from the posterior compartment by the pouch of Douglas (the rectouterine pouch) and the origin of the uterosacral ligaments. The uterosacral ligaments run from the cervix, around the rectum, to insert on the presacral fascia.

The posterior compartment is occupied by the rectum and is limited posteriorly by the sacral promontory.

The bony pelvis is lined on the inside by different muscle groups, and the muscles are covered with the endopelvic fascia. The endopelvic fascia forms two transverse layers of fascia that are attached laterally to the arcuate tendons. The anterior transverse layer is called the pubocervical fascia and extends from the pubis anteriorly to the cervix posteriorly, and it is also laterally attached to the arcuate tendons, which are formed by condensed areas of the lateral endopelvic pelvic fascia and run vertically. The pubocervical fascia supports the bladder and urethra anteriorly, and prevents the bladder from sagging into the vagina. The posterior transverse layer is called the rectovaginal septum and extends from the perineal body anteriorly to the cervix posteriorly. This layer supports the rectum posteriorly and prevents the rectum from bulging into the vagina.

The lateral limits of these compartments are lined by the arcuate tendons of the endopelvic fascia (also called the tendinous arc or white line), the iliac vessels, and the ureters, which cross over the tendons. The arcuate tendons, a linear thickening of the endopelvic fascia over the levator ani fascia, run in a straight line from the posterior aspect of the pubic bone to the ischial spine. These structures can be readily visualized depending on the amount of the surrounding adipose tissue.

The endopelvic fascia is visceral connective tissue found between the peritoneum and the parietal fascia covering the musculature of the pelvic basin. The pelvic basin is composed of a floor (the levator ani and coccygeus muscles), two sidewalls (the two obturator internus muscles), and a back wall (the piriformis muscles and sacrum). The front wall is the pubic symphysis. The endopelvic fascia forms sheets of visceral supporting tissue that fuse around viscera, arteries, and veins to form stronger sheaths. Also enveloped within these sheaths are visceral nerves, lymphatics, and adipose tissue.

The two main functions of the endopelvic fascia are to function as flexible conduits and physical supports for the visceral pelvic vasculature, visceral nerves, and lymph tissue; and to mechanically suspend the pelvic viscera (the bladder, cervix, vagina, and rectum) within the pelvis over the levator plate to secure pelvic visceral support. For instance, the cardinal ligaments not only surround and support the internal iliac vessels and uterine vessels, but also attach to the upper third of the vagina and cervix to position these structures horizontally over the levator plate for support. An understanding of the composition, function, and location of the endopelvic fascia facilitates retroperitoneal surgical dissections. Dissection in the proper plane between the endopelvic fascia and vessels allows the surgeon to safely perform lymphadenectomies.

In summary, the female pelvic viscera are supported by the pelvic floor and thickenings of the endopelvic fascia, including the cardinal and uterosacral ligaments.

The visible peritoneal folds include (from anterior to posterior) the round ligaments, the broad ligaments, the infundibulopelvic ligaments, and the uterosacral ligaments. Anterior to the uterus, a peritoneal recess (the anterior or vesicouterine pouch) is noted. A deeper posterior cul-de-sac, the pouch of Douglas, is found between the uterus and rectum.

Bladder and Urethra

The bladder is supported by a specific part of the endopelvic fascia called the pubocervical fascia. The pubocervical fascia extends from the pubis anteriorly to the cervix of the uterus posteriorly. The pubocervical fascia acts like a hammock to support the bladder in the correct position. The anterior (front) end of the pubocervical fascia supports the bladder neck and urethra, and the posterior (back) end of the pubocervical fascia supports the rest of the bladder.

Below the peritoneal recess that composes the vesicouterine fold, the bladder is connected to the upper vagina and cervix by areolar tissue, a plane that should be followed in cases of vaginal-sparing radical cystectomy. Development of this vesicovaginal space may be difficult and sometimes bloody. The bladder is stabilized at its neck, near the exit of the urethra, by the internal investing layer of the endopelvic fascia attached to the pubic bone. The remainder is free to move.

The space of Retzius is a potential avascular space with very vascular borders. It consists of an anterior compartment and two lateral compartments. The anterior compartment is bounded anteriorly by the pubic bone with the umbilicoprevesical fascia, and posteriorly by the endopelvic fascial capsule that surrounds the bladder. Contained within this endopelvic fascial capsule is the rich network of perivesical venous sinuses within deposits of areolar fat. Centrally over the urethra, just under the pubic arch, is the deep dorsal vein of the clitoris, which feeds into these venous channels. Therefore, the initial dissection of the anterior compartment of the space of Retzius should not be directed centrally where these vessels may be lacerated. The lateral compartment of the space of Retzius (the paravesical space) is bounded laterally by the obturator internus fascia and the obturator nerve artery and vein, just beneath the bony arcuate ridge of the ilium. The posterior border (toward the sacrum) is formed by the endopelvic fascial sheath around the internal iliac artery and vein and its anterior branches as they course toward the ischial spine. The floor of this lateral compartment is formed by the pubocervical fascia as it inserts into the arcuate tendons of the endopelvic fascia.

The arteries irrigating the bladder run in the depth of the pubocervical fascia and are composed of the superior, middle, and inferior vesical arteries that branch from the hypogastric, obturator, inferior gluteal, uterine, and vaginal arteries.

The female urethra is located behind the symphysis, embedded in the anterior vaginal wall; its direction is obliquely downward and forward. The urethra perforates the urogenital diaphragm, where it acquires longitudinal folds.

Vagina, Cervix, and Uterus

The vaginal longitudinal axis is toward the sacral promontory, and the cervix is suspended at the upper end, surrounded by the anterior, posterior, and lateral fornices. The upper two-thirds of the vagina is supported by the paravaginal fascia and the paracervical tissue (cardinal ligaments), the lower one-third by the perineal body.

The paracolpium and parametrium are the connective tissues that surround the vagina and uterus, respectively. In the mid vagina, the paracolpium fuses with the pelvic wall and fascia laterally. The cardinal ligaments (also called the transverse cervical ligaments of Mackenrodt) extend from the lateral margins of the cervix and upper vagina to the lateral pelvic walls. They are thickenings of the lowermost parts of the broad ligaments. Laterally, the cardinal ligaments are continuous with the connective tissue surrounding the hypogastric vessels. Medially, they are continuous with the paracolpium and the parametrium as well as with the connective tissue in the anterior vaginal wall (the pubocervical fascia).

The cardinal ligament contains the uterine artery traveling medially toward the lower uterine segment. Dissection of the pelvic sidewall naturally leads into this area, where the uterine artery branches from the internal iliac artery. The origin of the uterine artery may be laparoscopically identified by dissecting along the medial border of the obliterated umbilical artery while working backward toward the internal iliac artery. The medial branch is then identified as the uterine artery (Figure 2.14).

If the anterior vaginal wall is resected along with the specimen during radical cystectomy, laparoscopic staplers are usually able to control bleeders located in the depth of both the paracolpium (Figure 2.15). The distal third of the anterior wall of the vagina and the urethra are usually dissected from the perineum during radical cystectomy.

The posterior vaginal wall, below the cardinal ligaments (lower two thirds), is supported from the sides by the paracolpium, which is attached to the endopelvic fascia (referred to as rectovaginal fascia in this area) and the pelvic diaphragm. The anterior and posterior fascial layers unite along the sides of the vagina. The rectovaginal fascia is found mostly at the sides and is extremely thin in the midline of the vaginal wall. However, a posterior rectovaginal septum, consisting of fibromuscular elastic tissue, extending from the peritoneal reflection to the perineal body, has been described. The peritoneal cavity extends to the cranial part of the perineal body during fetal life, but becomes obliterated in early life. Its fused layers (Denonvilliers' fascia) probably

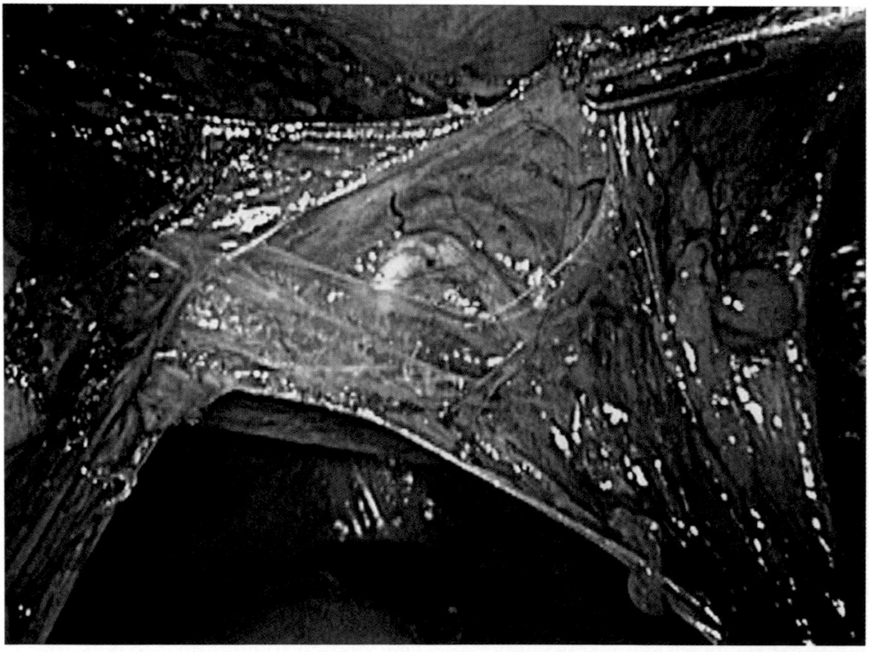

FIGURE 2.14. Right uterine artery surrounded by blue lymphatic channels after cervical injection of methylene blue for sentinel node mapping

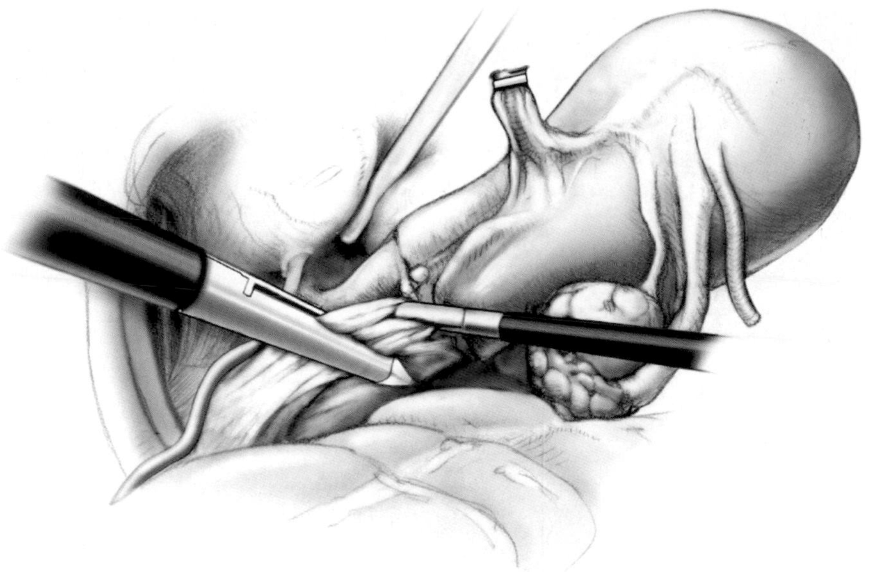

FIGURE 2.15. Vessels of left paracolpos exposed (shown controlled with laparoscopic stapler)

become part of the rectovaginal septum adherent to the undersurface of the posterior vaginal wall. This fascia forms the anterior margin of another potential space, the rectovaginal space. The rectovaginal septum, if intact and normal, permits independent mobility of the rectal and vaginal walls.

The uterine fundus is covered by peritoneum except in the lower anterior portion, where it is contiguous with the bladder and the peritoneum is reflected forming the vesicouterine fold, and laterally, where the folds of the broad ligaments are attached. The round ligaments are one of the most visible laparoscopic landmarks, curving from the lateral horns of the uterus to exit through the internal inguinal ring. These ligaments have only minor structural significance. Peritoneum covers the round ligaments and then descends on both sides to encompass the broad ligaments, which may be thought of as the mesentery of the uterus.

The uterus is supported by a thickening of the endopelvic fascia (visceral connective tissue found between the peritoneum and the parietal fascia covering the musculature of the pelvic brim) and fibromuscular tissue laterally at the base of the broad ligaments. The round ligaments and the uterovesical fold anteriorly provide weak uterine support.

The cervix is bound to the sacrum by the uterosacral ligaments or rectouterine ligaments. They run from the cervix, around the rectum, to insert into the presacral fascia over S2, S3, and S4. Anterior traction on the uterus places tension on the uterosacral ligaments, which makes them easier to identify (Figure 2.16). Near the cervix, the ureters are found just behind the peritoneum, just lateral to these ligaments.

Anatomic knowledge of the uterine and vaginal attachments is key during laparoscopic pelvic surgery in women. When the uterus is displaced to one side by gentle manipulation with a uterine manipulator or grasper, some of these attachments and the structures of the contralateral adnexa are spread out and more readily displayed. During radical cystectomy, the uterus is usually anteverted intraoperatively, and the initial peritoneotomy is made to identify the ureters posteriorly, which should be dissected all the way to the bladder wall, and then clipped and transected.

If the anterior vaginal wall is to be resected, then the peritoneum at the rectovesical pouch of Douglas is incised and dissection is continued to develop a short plane anterior to the rectum before the vagina is actually entered.

The cardinal and uterosacral ligaments are not directly important for continence but do play a role in supporting the base of the bladder when large cystoceles are surgically corrected. The vaginal arteries arise from the hypogastric artery below the level of the uterine artery and send branches to the vagina, bladder, and rectum.

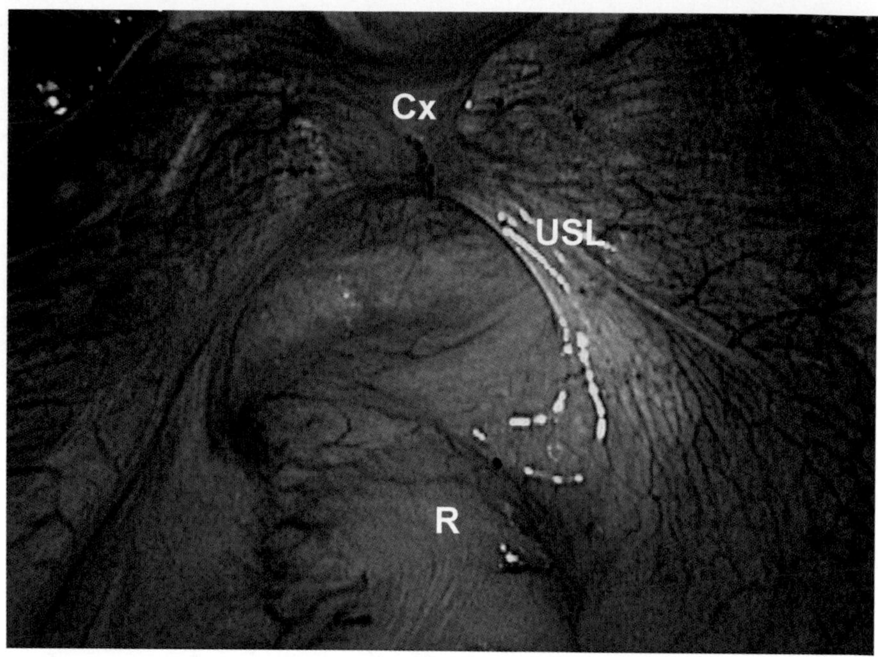

FIGURE 2.16. Posterior cul-de-sac and uterosacral ligaments (tubes and ovaries have been removed). Cx = cervix, R = rectum, USL = uterosacral ligament

Ovaries and Fallopian Tubes

The fallopian tubes (oviducts) arise from the superior portion of the lateral borders of the uterus, superior to the attachments of the round ligaments. The fallopian tubes are divided into interstitial, isthmic, ampullar, and fimbriated portions, with the latter opening into the peritoneal cavity. The other three portions are covered by peritoneum to form the upper borders of the broad ligament.

The ovaries are located on the posterior surface of the broad ligaments, inferior to the fallopian tubes. The ovaries are uncovered in the peritoneal cavity but are attached to the body wall via the suspensory ligament of the ovary. The ovaries are also attached to the uterus and fallopian tubes by the utero-ovarian and tubo-ovarian ligaments. The part of the broad ligament of the uterus that covers the ovary is known as the mesovarium. The vessels, nerves, and lymphatics enter the ovary at the point of attachment to the broad ligaments, the hilus. Lateral support of the ovaries is provided by the infundibulopelvic ligament, which contains the aforementioned pedicle and extends to the pelvic side wall (Figure 2.17). During radical cystectomy, control of both infundibulopelvic suspensory ligaments containing the ovarian vessels is key before dissection of the uterus and vagina (Figure 2.18).

Ureters

The abdominal part of the ureter lies on the medial part of the psoas muscle and is crossed obliquely by the ovarian vessels. The ureter enters the pelvis just superficial to either the distal part of the internal iliac vessels or the proximal section of the external iliac vessels, and just deep to the ovarian vessels, which are in the infundibulopelvic ligament. This entrance is located at the level of the pelvic brim overlying the sacroiliac juncture. In many patients, the course of the ureters in the pelvis can be seen as a peritoneal fold that extends from the iliac bifurcation to the posterior bladder wall, which facilitates their dissection.

The ureters travel in their own fascial lamina (Waldeyer's sheath), which is attached to the parietal peritoneum of the pelvic sidewall. In the patient placed in the dorsolithotomy position in preparation for laparoscopic surgery, the ureter courses almost horizontally and points toward the ischial spine.

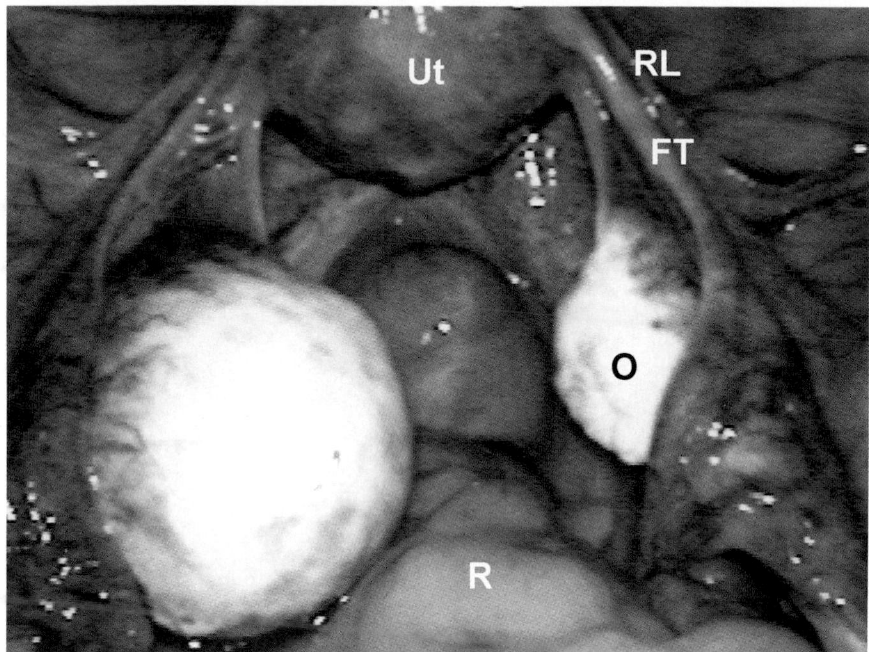

FIGURE 2.17. Adnexae and vasculature; note left ovarian cyst. FT = fallopian tube, O = ovary, R = rectum, RL = round ligament, Ut = uterus

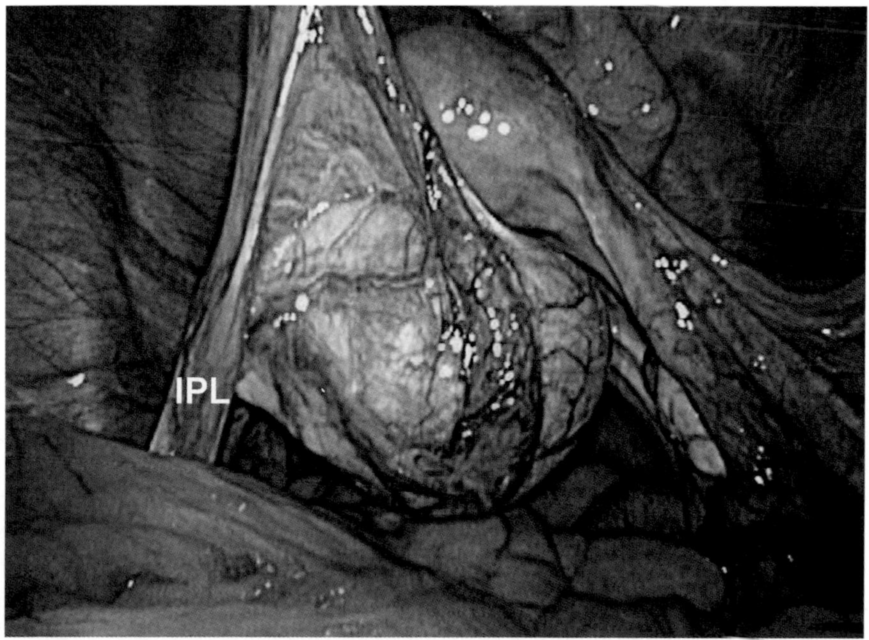

FIGURE 2.18. Left infundibulopelvic ligament; note left ovarian cyst. IPL = infundibulopelvic ligament

The ureter then passes just lateral to the uterosacral ligament, approximately 2 cm medial to the ischial spine. This area is just beneath the uterine artery, approximately 1.5-2 cm lateral to the side of the cervix. The ureter forms a "knee" turn at this point and travels medially and anteriorly to pass on the anterolateral aspect of the upper third of the vagina toward the bladder in its own fascia.

The ureter is accompanied by the uterine artery in its distal course. The uterine artery then crosses over the ureter and ascends following a tortuous route between the leaves of the broad ligament to enter the uterus laterally. The uterine artery finally unites with the ovarian artery on the side of the uterus to give off small branches to the uterus and round ligaments. An early branch of the uterine artery turns inferiorly on either side to form the cervical arteries. The blood supply of the ureter arises from the renal, ovarian, hypogastric, and inferior vesical arteries.

Four approaches have been described for the laparoscopic dissection of the ureters: medial, superior, lateral, and retrograde. The medial approach to the ureter is the simplest and is the approach that was initially used by most laparoscopic surgeons. It consists of sharply anteflexing the uterus to enable the ureter to be visualized through the peritoneum of the broad ligament in its natural position on the pelvic sidewall. A window is created in the peritoneum right above the ureter, allowing the infundibulopelvic pedicle to be safely divided. The limitations of this approach are that it cannot be used if pelvic pathology obscures the broad ligament, and it does not allow the pararectal space to be properly developed.

The superior approach entails identifying the ureter above the pelvic brim and then tracing it into the pelvis along the medial leaf of the broad ligament. A key maneuver is to pull the infundibulopelvic ligament medially to expose the underlying ureter. On the left side, the sigmoid colon must be mobilized first. Once the ureter has been identified and freed superiorly, it is then progressively reflected off the medial leaf of the broad ligament until the uterine vessels are reached (Figure 2.19).

The lateral approach to the ureter is similar to that used in open surgery and consists of opening the peritoneum of the pelvic sidewall, identifying the internal iliac artery, and opening the pararectal space by blunt dissection medial to the internal iliac artery.

Finally, the retrograde approach makes use of the umbilical ligament (obliterated hypogastric artery) based on the anatomic knowledge that dissection along the medial aspect of the obliterated umbilical artery toward the internal iliac artery in retrograde fashion allows the surgeon to locate the origin of the uterine artery. The umbilical ligament is bluntly dissected and traced proximally to where it joins the uterine artery to form the hypogastric artery. Blunt dissection proximal and medial to the uterine artery will open the pararectal space, the medial border of which is bounded by the ureter. The site at which the uterine arteries are divided and the extent to which the extraperitoneal spaces are developed and the ureters mobilized off the medial leaf of the broad ligament are tailored to the particular operation being performed.

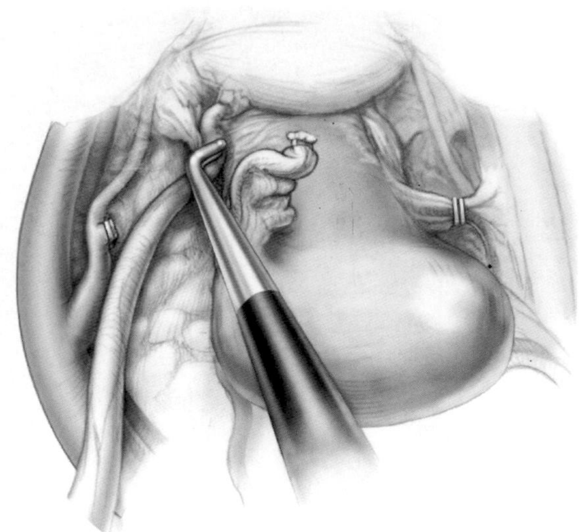

FIGURE 2.19. Left ureter unroofed from parametria

Vascular and Lymphatic Supplies

The major vascular and lymphatic supplies do not vary substantially from those of the male pelvis, except for the names and locations of the vessels irrigating the internal genitalia.

The iliac vessels originate as the common iliac arteries from the aorta at the L4 vertebral level and slightly to the left of midline. This is of particular importance when deciding the height of port placement to accomplish an extended pelvic lymph node dissection. An extended pelvic lymph node dissection is more difficult to accomplish if ports are placed too low.

Keeping in mind the high incidence of anatomic vascular variations, the hypogastric vessels are usually 3-4 cm long before they divide into anterior and posterior branches (Figure 2.20). The anterior branch provides the main blood supply to the bladder and forms the hemorrhoidal, obturator,

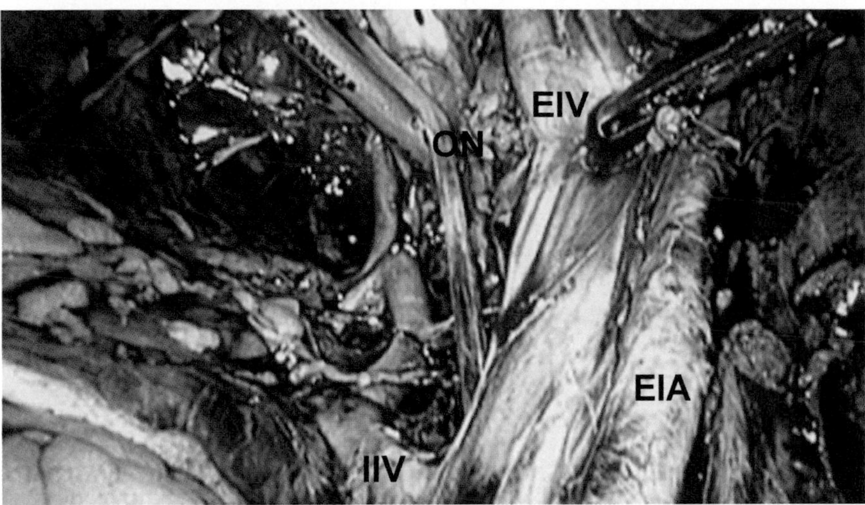

FIGURE 2.20. Right hypogastric vein; right external iliac vessels and obturator nerve are retracted laterally. EIA = external iliac artery, EIV = external iliac vein, IIV = internal iliac vein, ON = obturator nerve

internal pudendal, inferior gluteal, uterine, and vaginal arteries, as described previously.

The internal pudendal artery is the most caudal extension of the hypogastric artery and supplies the internal and external genitalia. The pudendal artery emerges from the pelvis between the piriformis and coccygeus muscles, crosses the ischial spine, and passes through the lesser sciatic foramen to enter the perineum. The artery traverses the lateral wall of the ischiorectal fossa and irrigates the erectile tissue of the vulva.

As in male anatomy, the lymphatics parallel the vascular channels in female anatomy. The lymphatic system is composed of multiple lymph nodes connected by an extensive network of intercommunicating capillaries and vessels. These structures are contained within the sheaths of endopelvic fascia, which also envelop the pelvic vasculature.

During radical cystectomy, all nodal tissue is cleared from the genitofemoral nerve laterally to the bladder wall medially, and from the distal common iliac artery superiorly to the lateral circumflex iliac vein and the node of Cloquet inferiorly. The obturator fossa is cleared of nodal tissue, preserving the obturator nerve (Figures 2.21 to 2.23). An extended lymph node dissection has also been recommended to include the common iliac, the presacral and the packages located around the distal 2-3 cm of the great vessels that compose the lower para-aortic and paracaval areas (Figure 2.24).

The "presacral" space is bounded anteriorly by the parietal peritoneum and posteriorly by the anterior longitudinal ligament and periosteum over the lowest two lumbar vertebrae and the promontory of the sacrum. The right lateral border is the right common iliac artery and the right ureter. The left lateral border is the left common iliac vein and left ureter, as well as the inferior mesenteric artery and vein traversing through the mesentery of the sigmoid colon. The middle sacral artery and a plexus of veins are attached superficial to the anterior longitudinal ligament. The endopelvic fascia envelopes fatty areolar tissue, visceral nerves, and lymphatic tissue in this space. When performing a "presacral" lymphadenectomy, the surgeon must excise all fatty areolar tissue in this area, ideally preserving the neural branches of the superior hypogastric plexus (see nerve supply).

Nerve Supply

The visceral nerves are enveloped within the endopelvic fascia and areolar fat. They enter the pelvis from the superior hypogastric plexus found in the presacral space. These nerves are multiple and fine, sometimes making them difficult to visualize, even with the laparoscope. The right and left hypogastric nerves then run along with their internal iliac arteries and ureters to enter their respective inferior hypogastric plexuses

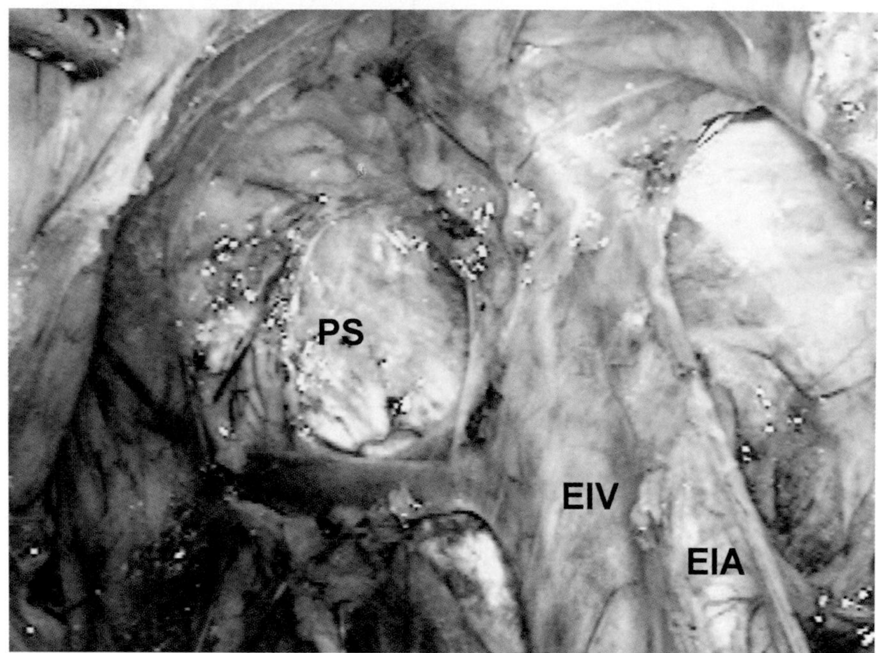

FIGURE 2.21. Left pelvic lymphadenectomy showing left circumflex iliac vein and obturator fossa. EIA = external iliac artery, EIV = external iliac vein, PS = pubic symphysis

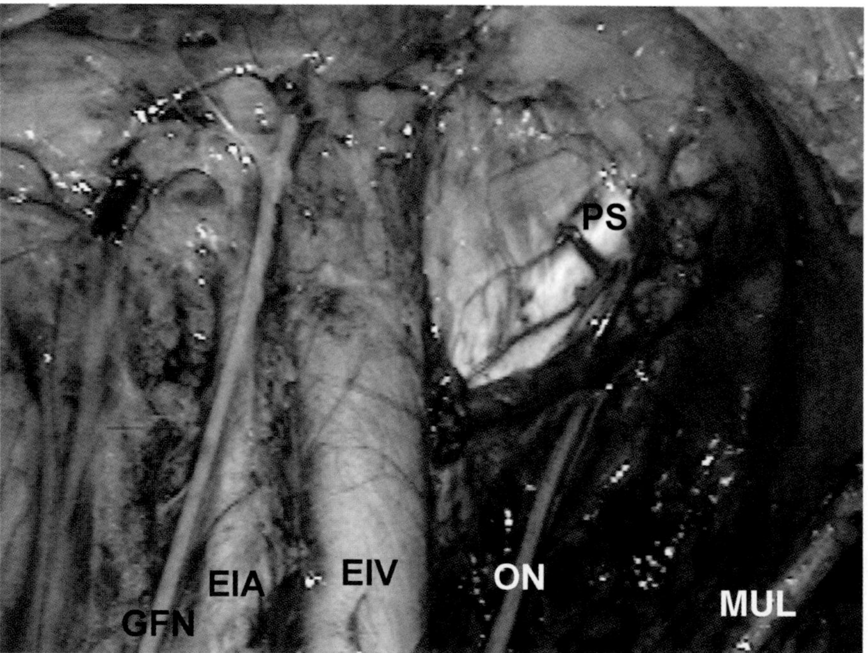

FIGURE 2.22. Right obturator fossa after lymphadenectomy; note presence of accessory obturator vein. EIA = external iliac artery, EIV = external iliac vein, GFN = genitofemoral nerve, ON = obturator nerve, PS = pubic symphysis, MUL = median umbilical ligament

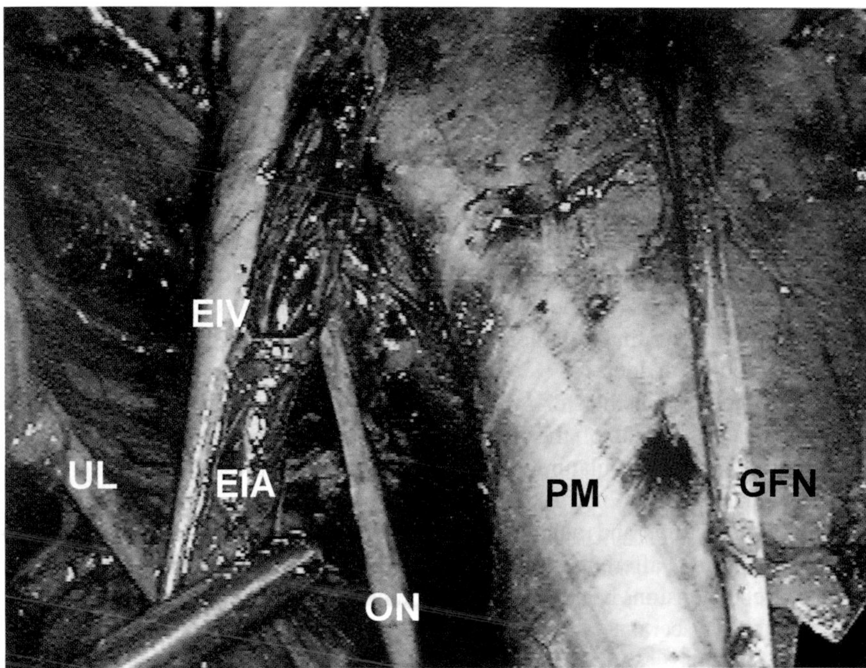

FIGURE 2.23. Lateral approach to right obturator space between external iliac vessels and psoas muscle. EIA = external iliac artery, EIV = external iliac vein, GFN = genitofemoral nerve, ON = obturator nerve, PM = psoas muscle, UL = median umbilical ligament

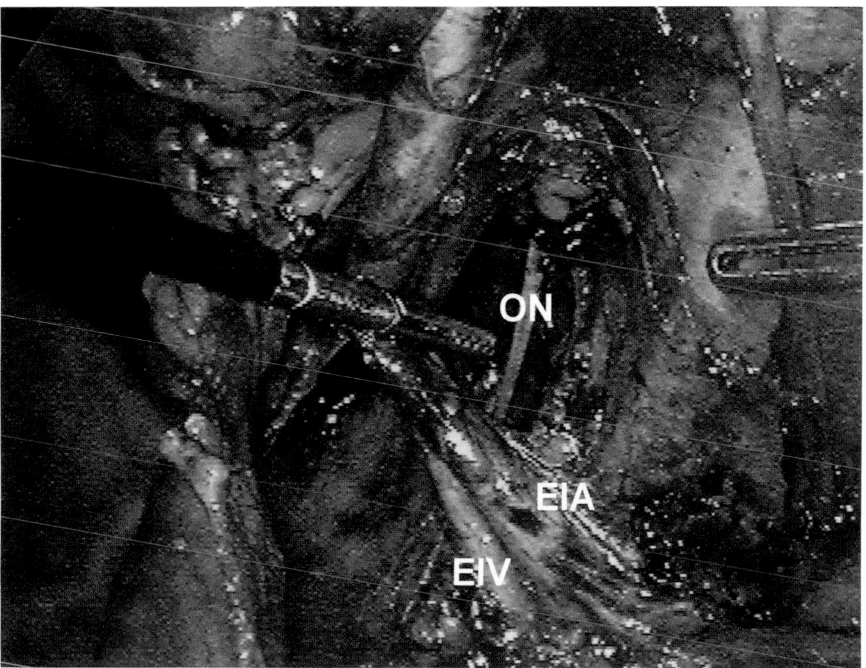

FIGURE 2.24. Common iliac and lower para-aortic and precaval lymphadenectomy (laparoscope is in suprapubic trocar site). EIA = external iliac artery, EIV = external iliac vein, ON = obturator nerve

hyperfunctioning adrenal tumors, such as aldosteronomas, which are generally small (85% weigh <10 g) and therefore ideally suited for laparoscopic excision. It is also the preferred option for adrenal incidentalomas requiring excision.

Laparoscopic adrenalectomy, whether unilateral or bilateral, can also be used to successfully treat Cushing's disease and syndrome. Since cushingoid patients have a propensity for poor wound healing and perioperative morbidity with open adrenalectomy, the minimally invasive approach may confer a significant advantage in this patient population.

The laparoscopic approach was once contraindicated for pheochromocytoma because of early concerns about perioperative cardiovascular complications; however, this procedure is now known to be safe and effective, potentially with less intraoperative hemodynamic fluctuations than are seen in open surgery.

Finally, although a small, radiologically organ-confined, noninfiltrating adrenal tumor with intact periadrenal fat planes can be excised laparoscopically, any large, irregular, and/or infiltrating adrenal tumor should be removed via open surgery with wide excision and en bloc lymphadenectomy.

Preoperative Evaluation and Patient Preparation

In addition to routine preoperative testing, patients undergoing laparoscopic adrenalectomy should undergo a thorough evaluation for adrenal biochemical activity, typically in conjunction with an endocrinologist or hypertension specialist. Preferred preoperative imaging comprises volume-rendered thin-slice 3-D reconstructed CT scanning, which provides the necessary detailed anatomic information regarding the vascularity and spatial relationships of the adrenal mass and adjacent blood vessels (eg, aorta, inferior vena cava, superior mesenteric artery, and renal vessels).

Endocrinologic Preparation

Hormonal and metabolic sequelae associated with adrenal tumors must be specifically identified and corrected preoperatively to ensure smooth patient outcomes.

In patients with a pheochromocytoma, preoperative preparation includes calcium channel blockade and expansion of the intravascular space with vigorous hydration and liberal salt intake. Alpha-adrenergic antagonists and beta-blockers are used secondarily and selectively. Patients with an aldosteronoma are treated preoperatively with potassium-sparing diuretics and potassium supplementation to achieve normal blood pressure. In patients with Cushing's disease, steroid replacement for perioperative stress is necessary and gradually weaned after surgery.

General Preparation

If the patient is taking anticoagulants, they are discontinued well in advance of surgery. All patients are admitted on the morning of surgery, except those with pheochromocytoma, who are admitted the day before surgery for intravenous hydration. To prepare the bowels, the patient is instructed to ingest magnesium citrate on the evening prior to surgery. Patients with pheochromocytoma also undergo invasive intraoperative hemodynamic monitoring.

Intraoperative Considerations

During laparoscopic adrenalectomy, the adrenal gland parenchyma must not be grasped with laparoscopic forceps. The adrenal gland is friable and prone to fracture if grasped firmly, potentially leading to local tumor spillage and continuous oozing and hemorrhage. Furthermore, the edge of the adrenal gland is circumferentially surrounded by a delicate arborizing arcade of blood vessels, which are likely to bleed if disrupted, considerably hampering intraoperative visualization. As a general rule, laparoscopic adrenalectomy should be performed from outside the periadrenal fat, which is a safer and less vascular plane, with more well-defined blood vessels that lend themselves to individual control.

Transperitoneal Technique

Patient Positioning

The patient is secured in a 45° to 60° lateral flank position, with the kidney rest partially elevated and the table mildly flexed to increase the space between the costal margin and the iliac crest. Because increased or prolonged lateral flexion can result in significant neuromuscular sequelae, the table should be straightened after achieving pneumoperitoneum and operative exposure of the adrenal gland. Although it is important to limit the degree of lateral flexion in either transperitoneal or retroperitoneal renal and adrenal surgery, table flexion is more important for obtaining initial access in the retroperitoneal approach. The patient's arms and legs are maintained in a neutral position, and all dependent bony prominences are carefully padded with egg-crate foam and blankets. An axillary roll is used to guard against brachial plexus injury, and the arms are secured in a double armboard. Intravenous lines, arterial lines, and blood pressure cuffs are placed in or on the nondependent arm.

Transperitoneal Right Adrenalectomy

Port Placement

After pneumoperitoneum has been established using a Veress needle, 4 ports are inserted. A right-hand working port (10 or 12 mm) is placed just under the costal margin, at the lateral edge of the rectus abdominis; a camera port (10 mm) is placed 3 fingerbreadths below the costal margin along the lateral margin of the rectus muscle; a 5-mm port is placed at the lateral border of the rectus muscle at the level of the umbilicus; and a 5-mm port is placed near the xiphoid for cephalad retraction of the liver. (Figure 3.1)

Cephalad Retraction of the Liver and Exposure of the Vena Cava

The liver is tautly retracted anterosuperiorly, using the shaft of a 5-mm laparoscopic locking clamp (e.g., an Allis clamp). The locking clamp is attached to the lateral parietal peritoneum high in the region of the rib cage, thus creating a system that maintains constant liver retraction without requiring any manual retraction. Because the 5-mm port for liver retraction is placed rather high, it is critical to ensure that the shaft of the locking clamp does not injure the liver or gall bladder. Occasionally, peritoneal bands tethering the liver need to be released to achieve appropriate liver retraction, which then provides excellent visualization of the upper pole kidney and adrenal gland, both of which are covered by Gerota's fascia.

A generous horizontal peritoneotomy incision is made parallel and adjacent to the inferior liver edge, exposing the immediately underlying adrenal gland and suprarenal inferior vena cava. Typically, significant mobilization of the right colon and duodenum is not required to obtain adequate exposure of the adrenal gland. However, the curve of the duodenum may overlie the inferior vena cava and renal hilum, requiring careful identification and medial mobilization (Figure 3.2).

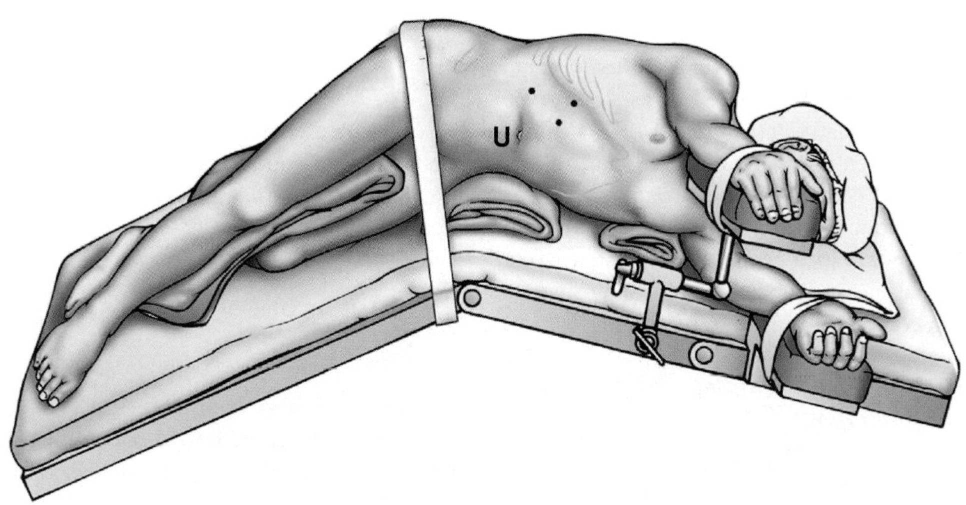

FIGURE 3.1. Transperitoneal right adrenalectomy. Patient positioning and port placement

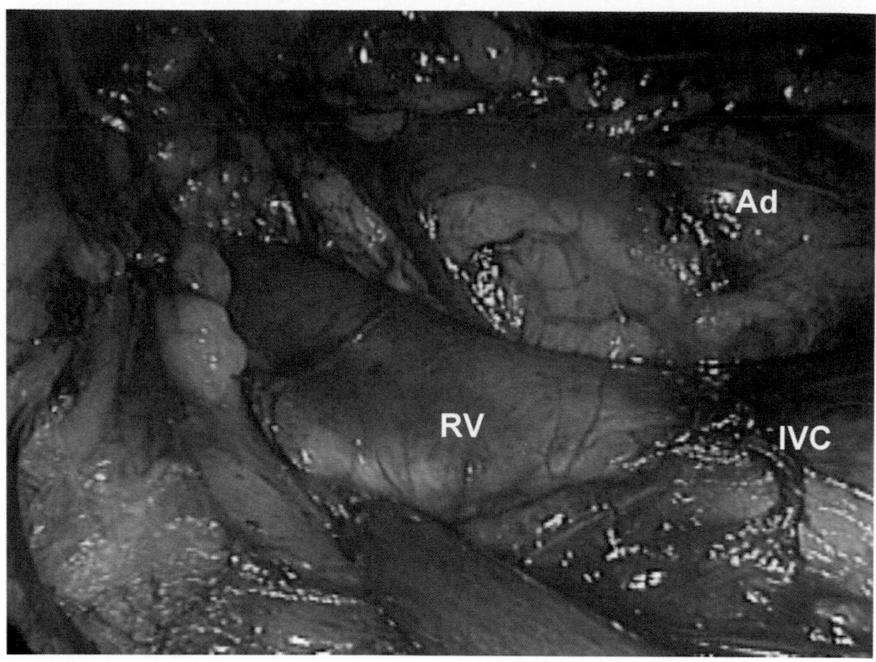

FIGURE 3.2. Transperitoneal right adrenalectomy. After mobilization of the duodenum, the inferior vena cava (IVC) is exposed and the renal vein (RV) dissected. The adrenal mass (Ad) is localized superior to the renal vein and lateral to the inferior vena cava

Dissection of the Adrenal Gland and Control of the Adrenal Vein

The adrenal gland is carefully mobilized laterally from the inferior vena cava. Multiple small aortic branches (transversely oriented) and renal hilar branches (obliquely oriented) to the adrenal gland are clipped and divided during this dissection. The dissection is continued cephalad until the main adrenal vein at the superomedial aspect of the adrenal gland is identified (Figure 3.3). This vein is thin-walled, and extreme care must be taken during its mobilization (Figure 3.4). The adrenal vein is securely clipped with locking clips and then divided. On rare occasions, such as in the circumstance of a larger adrenal mass, a laparoscopic stapler may be required to control the right adrenal vein.

Circumferential Mobilization of the Adrenal Gland

The adrenal gland is carefully dissected along the avascular plane immediately adjacent to the parenchyma of the upper pole of the kidney. Blood vessels derived from the renal hilum are controlled inferomedially, and care must be taken not to compromise an occasional aberrant artery in the upper renal pole. The adrenal gland is then dissected from the diaphragm after securing the inferior phrenic vascular supply.

Specimen Entrapment and Extraction

The excised adrenal gland is entrapped in an impermeable 10-mm endoscopic bag and extracted intact through an appropriately minimal extension of the inferior pararectal port site.

Transperitoneal Left Adrenalectomy

Port Placement

Typically, a 3-port approach is used, with port placement mirroring that of the right side template, except for the absence of the liver retraction port. Occasionally, an additional port may be

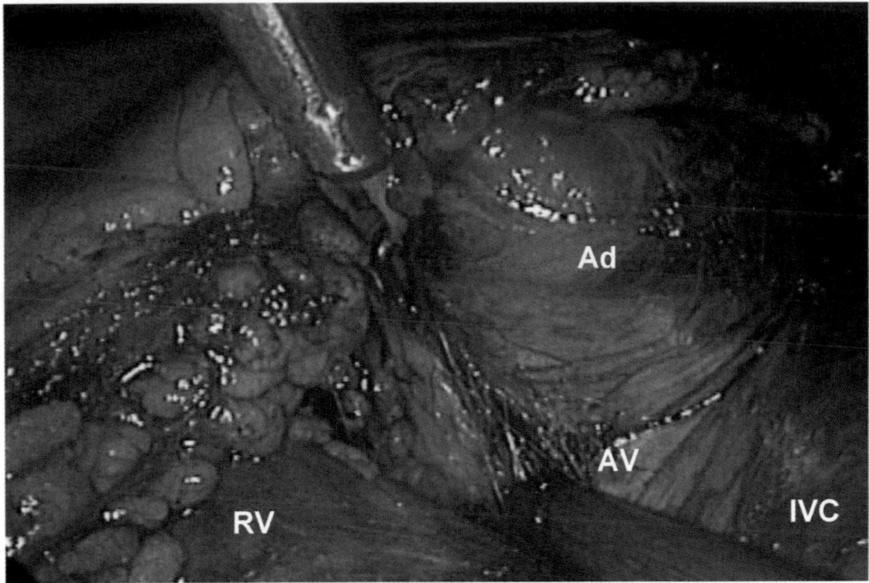

FIGURE 3.3. Transperitoneal right adrenalectomy. Mobilization of the adrenal mass (Ad) to gain access to the adrenal vein (AV). RV = renal vein, IVC = inferior vena cava

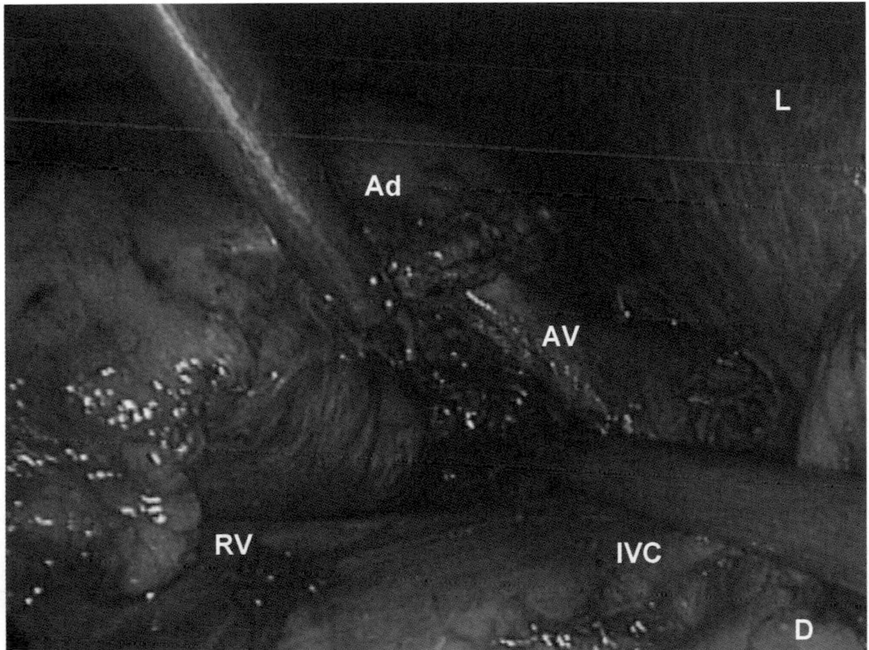

FIGURE 3.4. Transperitoneal right adrenalectomy. Mobilization of the adrenal mass (Ad) to gain access to the adrenal vein (AV). RV = renal vein, IVC = inferior vena cava, L = liver, D = duodenum

required for medial retraction of the descending colon and pancreas, especially in an obese patient (Figure 3.5).

Mobilization of the Colon and Spleen

In contrast to the right side, transperitoneal left adrenalectomy requires formal mobilization of the splenic flexure, left colon, spleen, and pancreatic tail. The line of Toldt is incised, and the colon, spleen, and tail of the pancreas are mobilized medially to expose the left adrenal gland (Figures 3.6 and 3.7).

Control of the Left Adrenal Vein

The main left renal vein is a main landmark. If it is difficult to recognize it immediately and approach it directly after the colon has been mobilized, the left gonadal vein can be traced to the left renal vein. Dissection along the cephalad aspect of the renal vein brings the left adrenal vein into view, which is carefully dissected, clipped, and divided (as above) (Figures 3.8 and 3.9). Care should be exercised during this maneuver to prevent injury to an upper pole branch of the renal artery, which may lie immediately posterior to the main left adrenal vein.

Mobilization of the Adrenal Gland

Once the main left adrenal vein is secured, the adrenal gland is systematically mobilized circumferentially—dissecting around the adrenal capsule—in a plane that can contain some fat in continuity with the perirenal fat (Figure 3.10). First, the medial border of the adrenal gland is freed by clipping the aortic branches, keeping the psoas muscle in clear and constant horizontal view. Then the superomedial edge of the adrenal gland is mobilized by controlling the inferior phrenic vessels, eventually using locking clips according to their size (otherwise accurate bipolar coagulation can safely be used). The inferior aspect of the adrenal gland is mobilized from the main renal artery and vein in a slow, deliberate fashion, maintaining hemostasis at all times (Figure 3.11). Laterally, the adrenal gland is separated from the upper pole of the left kidney. Once again we should emphasize that care must be taken not to inadvertently injure an upper pole renal artery that could not have been recognized preoperatively. The freed adrenal gland is then entrapped immediately and extracted intact.

Retroperitoneal Technique

Patient Positioning

Retroperitoneoscopic adrenalectomy is performed with the patient positioned in the conventional full-flank position. The retroperitoneal approach requires elevation of the kidney and lateral flexion during the initial access, but once access has been attained and ports adequately positioned, table

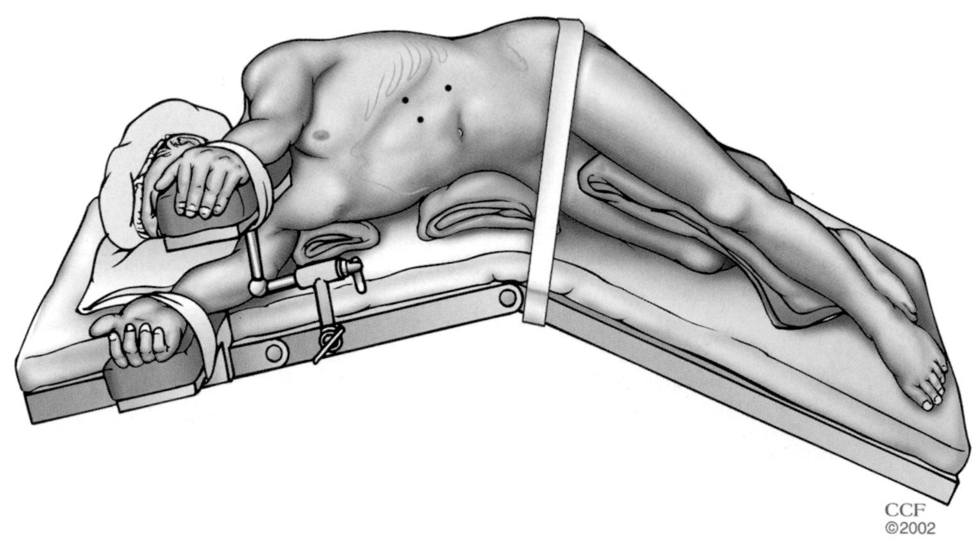

FIGURE 3.5. Transperitoneal left adrenalectomy. Patient positioning mirrors the right side template. Only 3 ports are used, unless retraction of the descending colon and pancreas is necessary

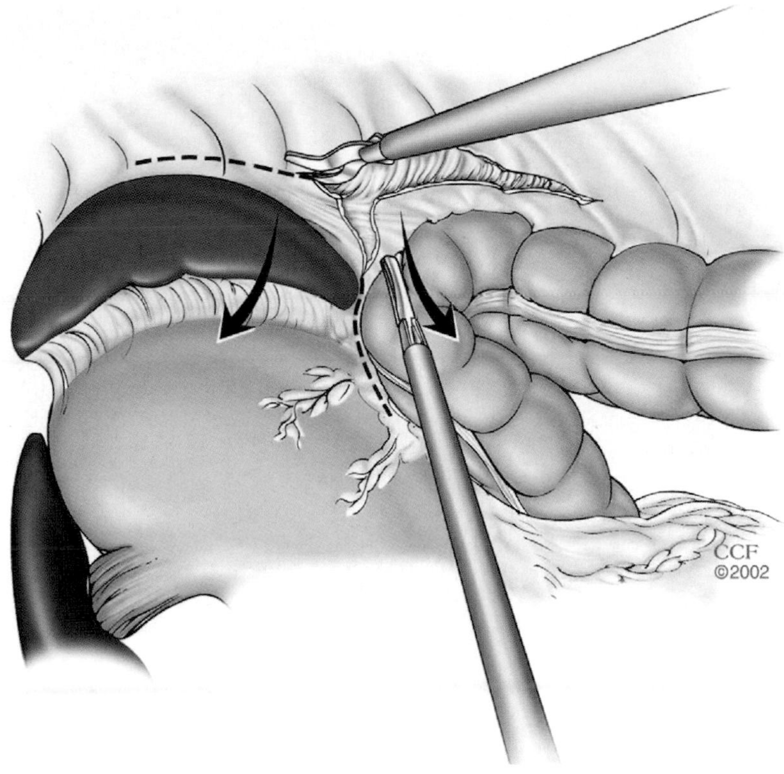

FIGURE 3.6. Transperitoneal left adrenalectomy. The spleen must be fully mobilized and flipped over its pedicle; then the splenocolic ligaments and line of Toldt are incised

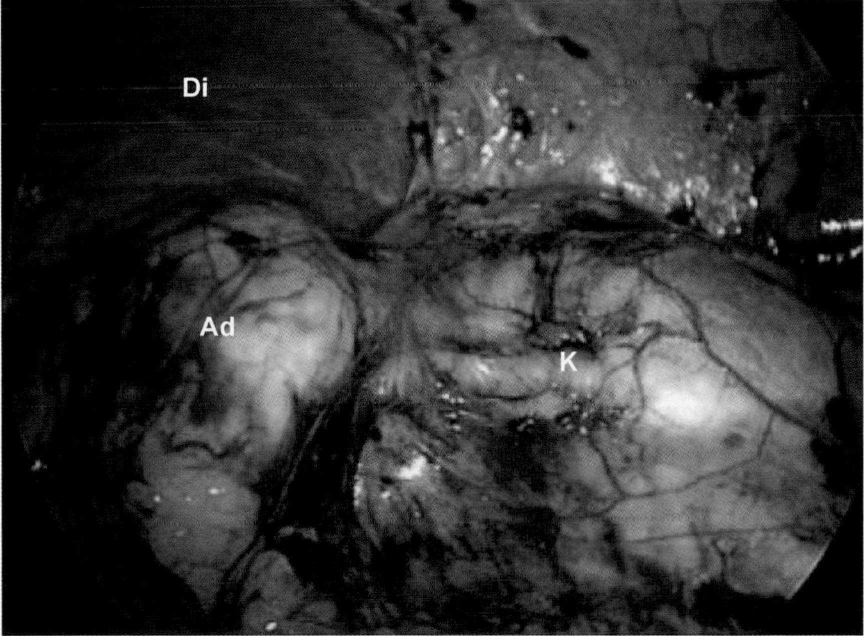

FIGURE 3.7. Transperitoneal left adrenalectomy. After the spleen and descending colon have been mobilized, the kidney (K) and the adrenal mass (Ad) are clearly exposed. Di = diaphragm

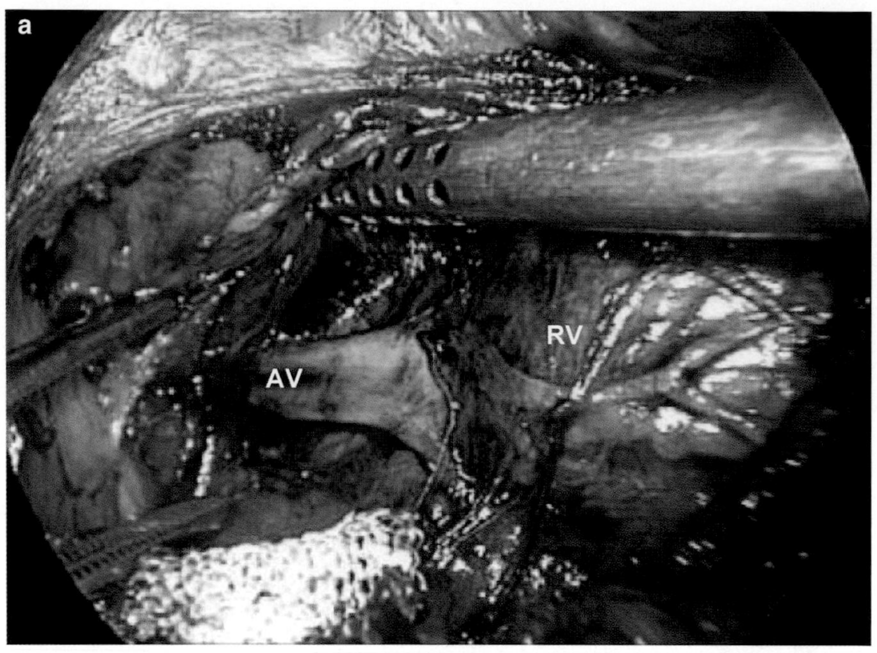

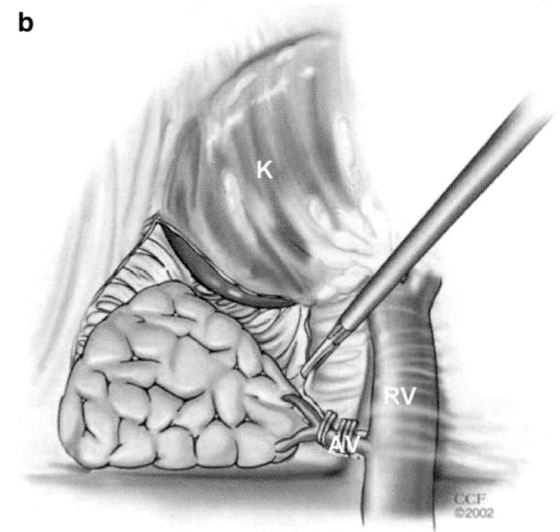

FIGURE 3.8. **(a)** Transperitoneal left adrenalectomy. Dissection of the upper aspect of the renal vein (RV) exposes the adrenal vein (AV). **(b)** Transperitoneal left adrenalectomy. Dissection of the left renal vein (RV) exposes the left adrenal vein (AV). The kidney (K) is not mobilized

flexion is reversed to minimize neuromuscular sequelae. Extreme flexion is not called for because it adds minimally, if at all, to the actual intraoperative exposure and dissection.

Retroperitoneal Access and Port Placement

Patient positioning and port placement are identical for right or left adrenalectomy (Figures 3.12 and 3.13). A 1.5-cm horizontal incision is made at the

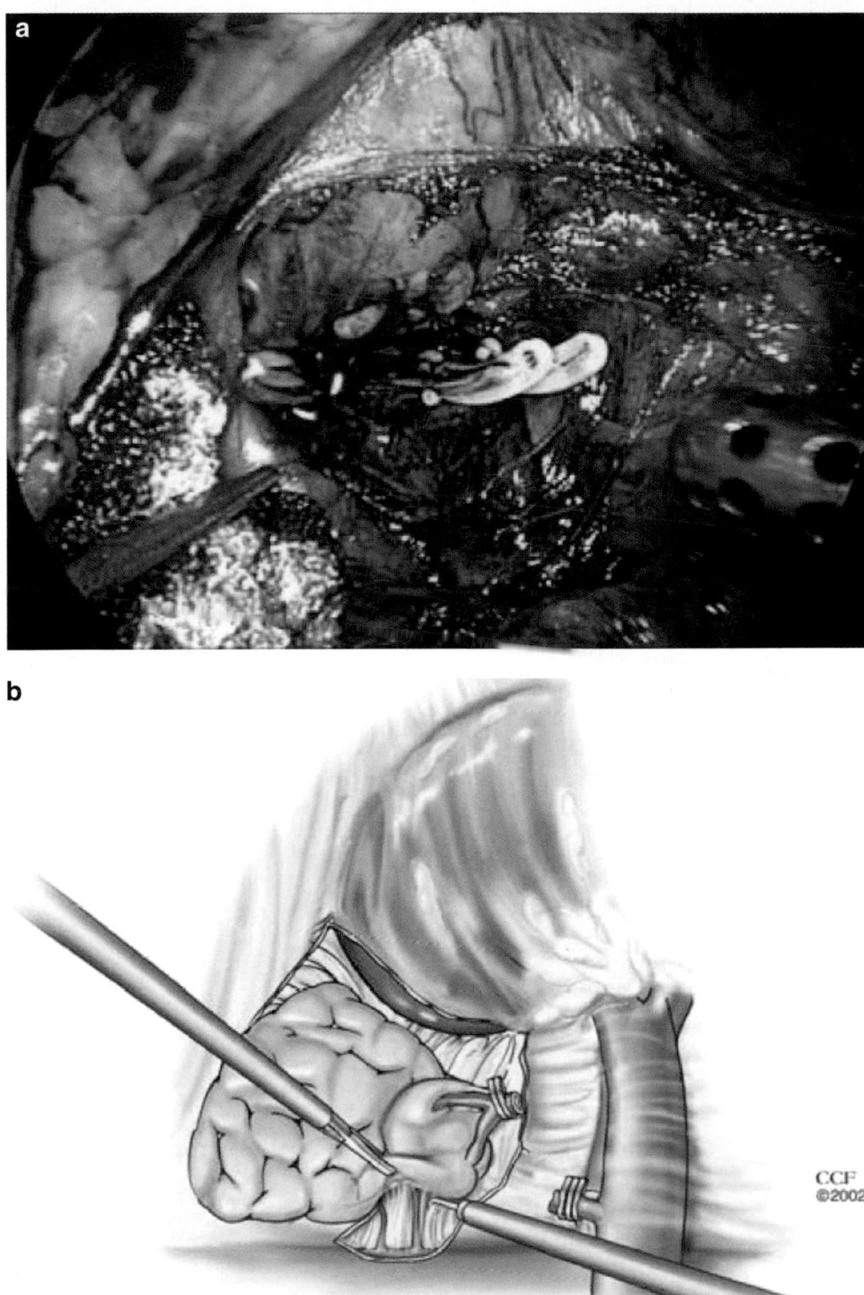

FIGURE 3.9. **(a)** Transperitoneal left adrenalectomy. Before the adrenal mass is mobilized, the adrenal vein is clipped and transected. **(b)**Transperitoneal left adrenalectomy. After the adrenal vein has been transected, the adrenal gland (embedded in the periadrenal fat) is dissected

tip of the 12th rib, and the flank muscle fibers are separated using 2 S retractors to visualize the whitish thoracolumbar fascia. A small 1-cm incision is then created with the tip of an electrocautery blade. Index finger dissection is performed to digitally perforate the thoracolumbar fascia and enter the

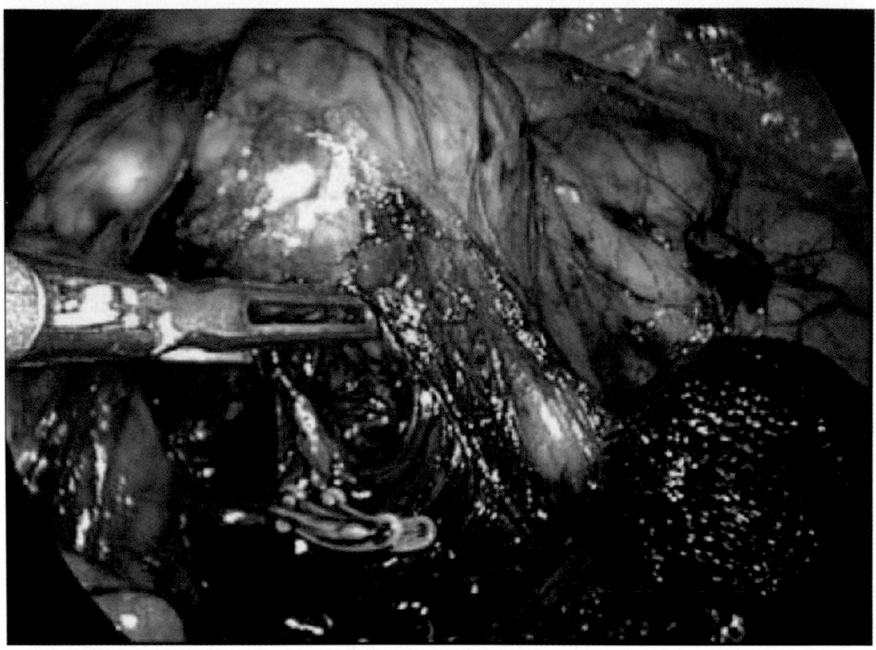

FIGURE 3.10. Transperitoneal left adrenalectomy. Mobilization of the adrenal mass and the adrenal gland from the surrounding periadrenal fascia and fat

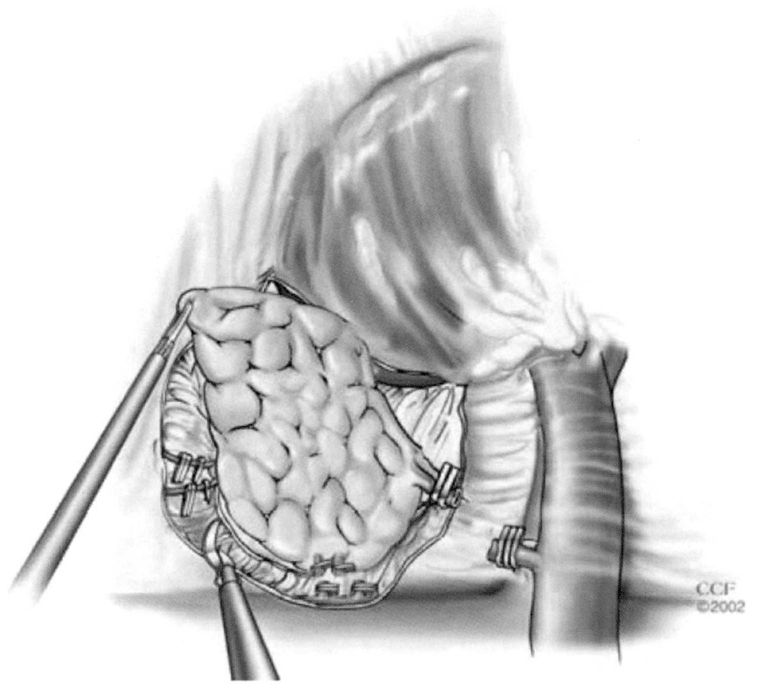

FIGURE 3.11. Transperitoneal left adrenalectomy. After the adrenal gland has been mobilized, small medial arteries are controlled by bipolar coagulation or clips

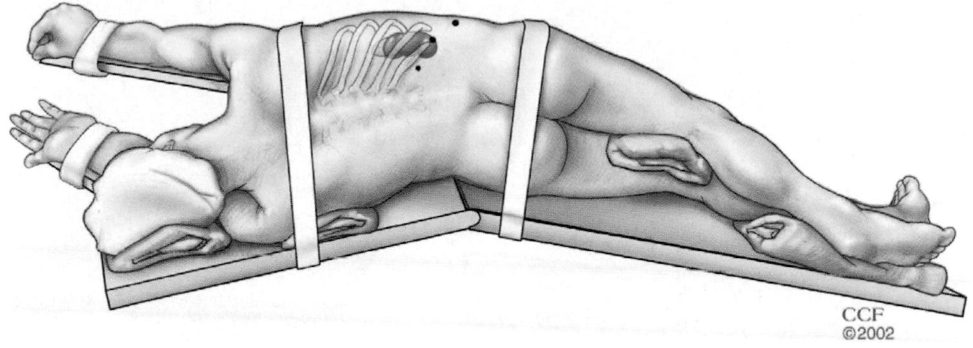

FIGURE 3.12. Retroperitoneoscopic right adrenalectomy. Patient positioning and port placement. A 3-port approach is used, but occasionally a fourth port may be required for retraction

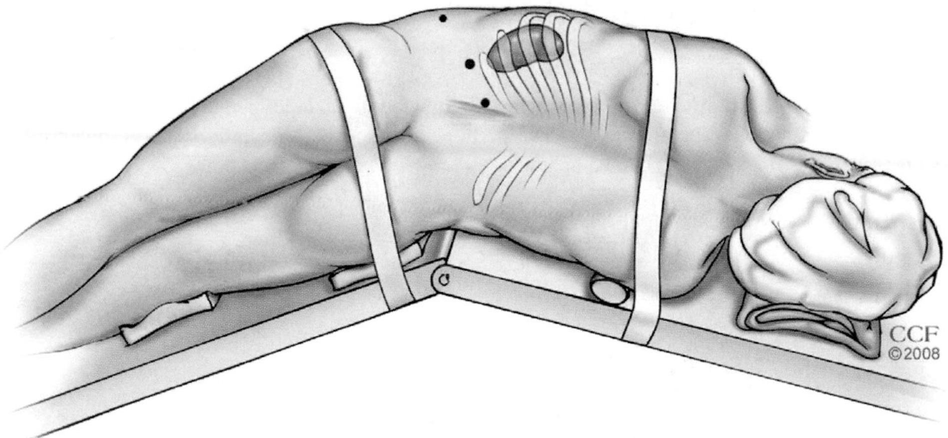

FIGURE 3.13. Retroperitoneoscopic left adrenalectomy. Patient positioning and port placement

retroperitoneum (Figure 3.14). This creates a space anterior to the psoas muscle/fascia and posterior to Gerota's fascia.

The retroperitoneal space can be developed atraumatically by balloon inflation to 800 cc. Six to eight pumps of a sphygmomanometer bulb will instill approximately 150 cc of air into the balloon (20 cc/pump). Retracting the shaft of the balloon dilator presses the balloon against the undersurface of the anterior abdominal wall. An additional 30 pumps of the sphygmomanometer bulb should be sufficient to create the retroperitoneal space. This maneuver ensures that the entire peritoneal reflection is mobilized medially, without any overhanging peritoneal shelf (Figure 3.15).

Secondary balloon inflation in the upper retroperitoneum may be necessary during a retroperitoneoscopic adrenalectomy. This is done by manually directing the shaft of the balloon dilator cephalad. A 10-mm port is secured at this skin incision and pneumoperitoneum achieved to 15–20 mmHg. After verifying appropriate retroperitoneal access, an anterior port (10 or 12 mm) is placed approximately 3 or 4 fingerbreadths cephalad to the anterior superior iliac spine (Figure 3.16), and a posterior port (10 or 12 mm) is placed under laparoscopic visualization in

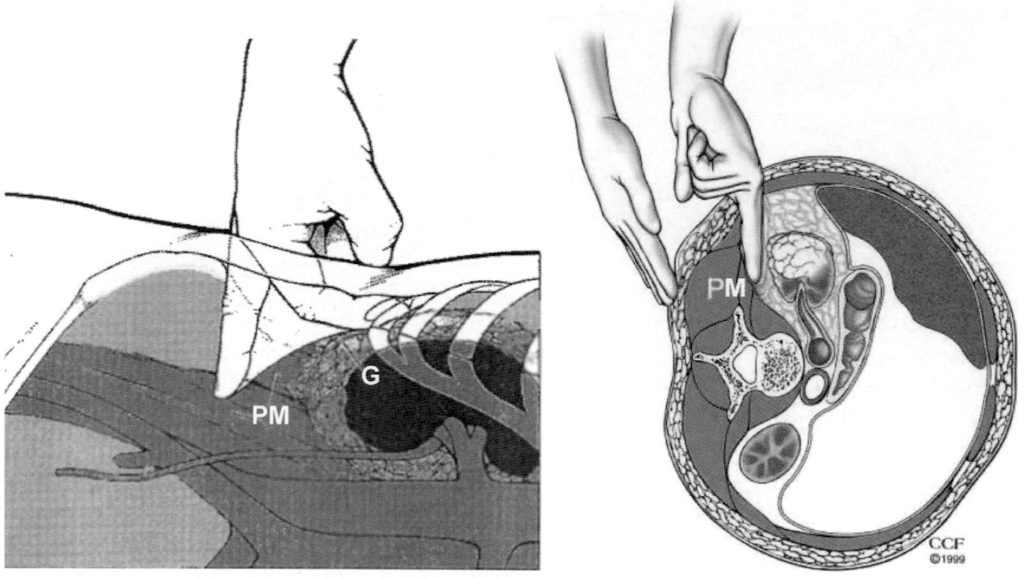

FIGURE 3.14. Finger dissection of the retroperitoneal space (right side). An index finger is placed in the space between the lumbar aponeurosis and Gerota's fascia (1). The peritoneum is pushed medially (2). The quadratus lumborum muscle and the (3) psoas muscle (PM) can be palpated

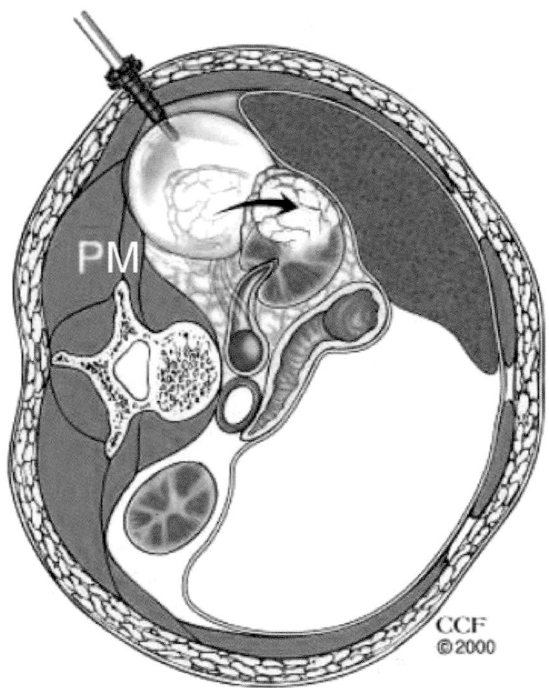

FIGURE 3.15. Balloon dissection of the retroperitoneum. Inflating the balloon between the psoas muscle (PM) and the kidney displaces the latter anteromedially *(arrow)*, allowing direct access to the renal hilum. The dilation process can be monitored laparoscopically through the transparent balloon

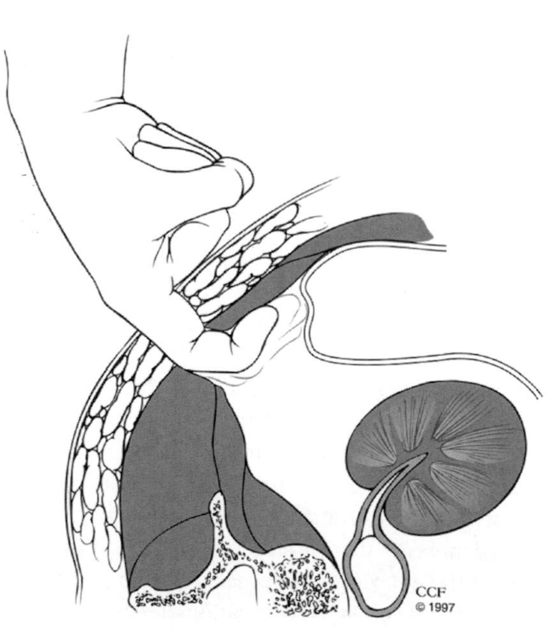

FIGURE 3.16. Retroperitoneoscopic approach. The lateral peritoneal reflection is mobilized before the secondary ports are inserted. One finger is inserted through the primary port site at the tip of the 12th rib

the costovertebral angle between the erector spinae muscle and the undersurface of the 12th rib.

Retroperitoneoscopic Right Adrenalectomy

Identification of the Renal Artery and Suprarenal Inferior Vena Cava

Right adrenalectomy begins with identification of the main right renal artery (vertical, forceful, bounding pulsations can be observed) (Figure 3.17). Next, the inferior vena cava, superior to the renal artery, is identified by its horizontal, wavy, gentler undulating pulsations. The fibroadipose tissue overlying the vena cava is carefully dissected. During this dissection, multiple small aortic and renal hilar branches to the adrenal gland are controlled. Dissection carefully continues cephalad along the surface of the vena cava.

Control of the Main Adrenal Vein

The main adrenal vein, identified high under the liver edge as it enters the posterolateral aspect of the vena cava, is clipped and divided. Extreme care must be taken, since any caval hemorrhage may be difficult to control and could require free-hand retroperitoneoscopic suturing (Figure 3.18).

Mobilization of the Adrenal Gland

The superior aspect of the adrenal gland is mobilized, dissecting it from the inferior surface of the diaphragm. The inferior phrenic supply to the adrenal gland is clipped and divided, and its anterior surface is subsequently mobilized from the peritoneal envelope. The inferior aspect of the adrenal gland is mobilized from the upper renal pole, and small vessels arising from the renal hilum are controlled. During this dissection, the surgeon should be aware of the possibility of an aberrant upper-pole renal artery.

Retroperitoneoscopic Left Adrenalectomy

Identification of the Left Renal Artery and Main Left Adrenal Vein

Similar to the procedure for right adrenalectomy, the initial step is identification of the main left renal artery (Figure 3.19). Dissection around the

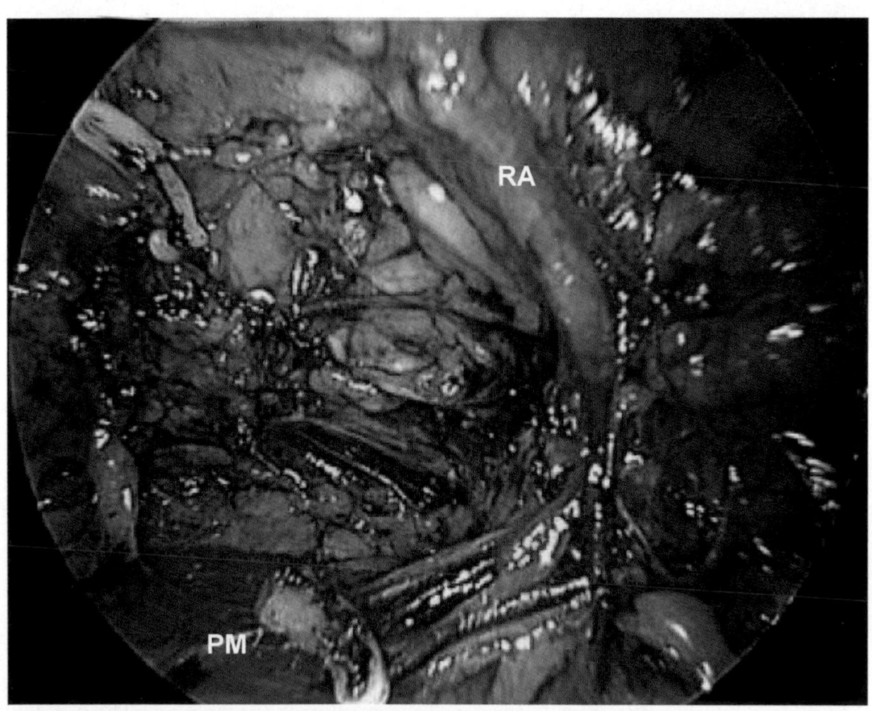

FIGURE 3.17. Retroperitoneoscopic right adrenalectomy. The first landmark is the identification of the renal artery, which is rising vertically. PM = psoas muscle, RA = renal artery

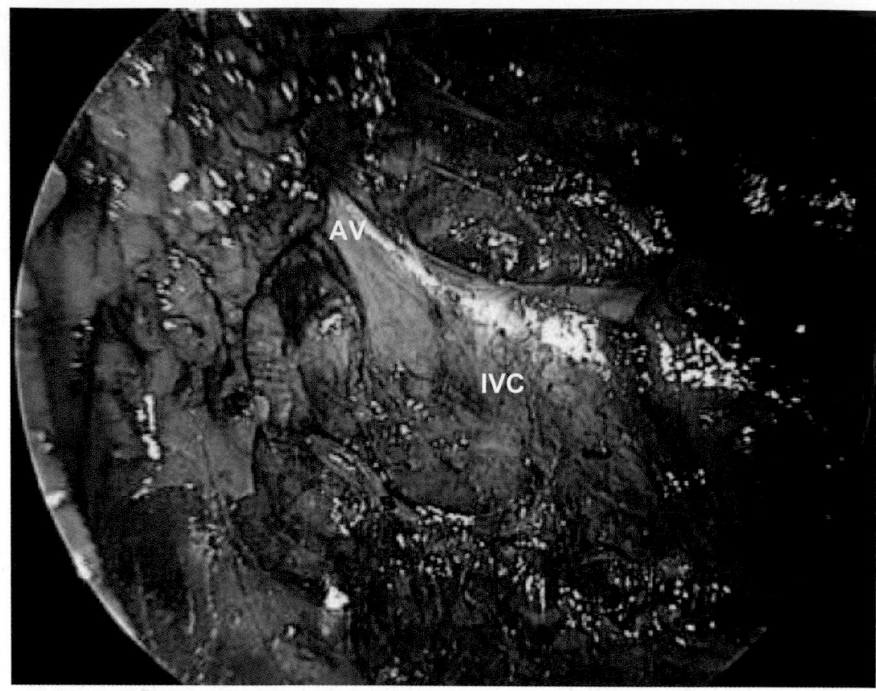

FIGURE 3.18. Retroperitoneoscopic right adrenalectomy. Dissection of the inferior vena cava (IVC) leads to the adrenal vein (AV), which will be clipped before mobilizing the adrenal mass and gland

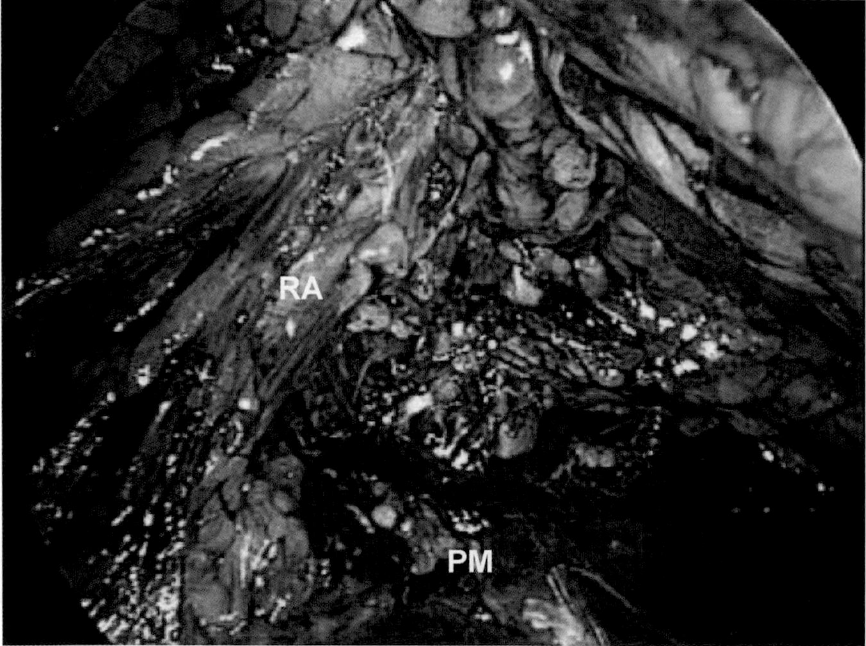

FIGURE 3.19. Retroperitoneoscopic left adrenalectomy. After the retroperitoneal space has been developed, the left renal artery (RA) is clearly visible. The space is developed superiorly to the renal hilum. The psoas muscle (PM) is kept horizontal throughout the procedure

superior aspect of the renal artery may bring the left adrenal vein into view (Figure 3.20). After the adrenal vein is identified, it is dissected, clipped, and divided.

Mobilization of the Medial Border of the Adrenal Gland

Multiple small aortic branches to the adrenal gland are also clipped and divided. This mobilizes the medial border of the adrenal gland from the aorta.

Mobilization of the Upper Renal Pole

Because most of the left adrenal gland is situated along the medial aspect of the upper renal pole, lateral and caudal mobilization of the upper renal pole is essential to gain access to the adrenal gland. Following adequate mobilization and lateral retraction of the upper pole kidney, the adrenal gland is carefully dissected from the kidney surface (Figure 3.21). Sparing the fascia that covers the adrenal gland will help protect the gland and also the tumor from being breached inadvertently. During the dissection the surgeon must be on the lookout for an accessory upper pole renal artery. Occasionally, the main adrenal vein cannot be identified earlier during the dissection; if so, it will be possible to identify and control it at this stage of the procedure.

Mobilization of the Adrenal Gland

The anterior surface of the adrenal gland is bluntly dissected from the undersurface of the peritoneum. If there is a communicating vein from the inferior phrenic vein to the main adrenal vein, it will probably course along the anteromedial aspect of the adrenal gland. The superior edge of the adrenal gland is mobilized from the undersurface of the diaphragm, while the inferior phrenic vessels are carefully controlled

Postoperative Care

The management of patients after adrenalectomy varies widely according to the nature of the disease, with a specific emphasis for hyperfunctioning tumors.

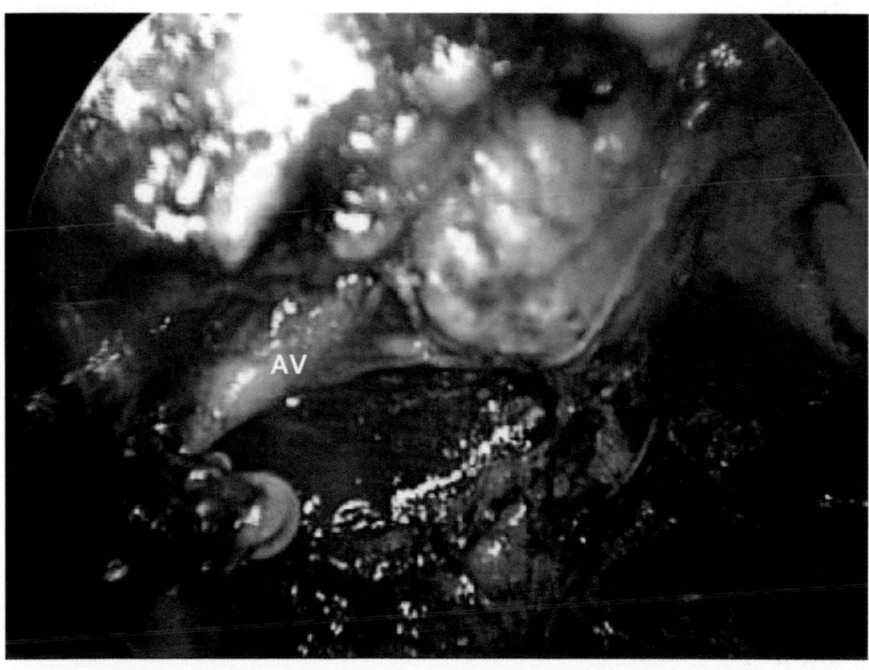

FIGURE 3.20. Retroperitoneoscopic left adrenalectomy. The dissection of the renal hilum superiorly exposes the adrenal vein, which is circumferentially dissected

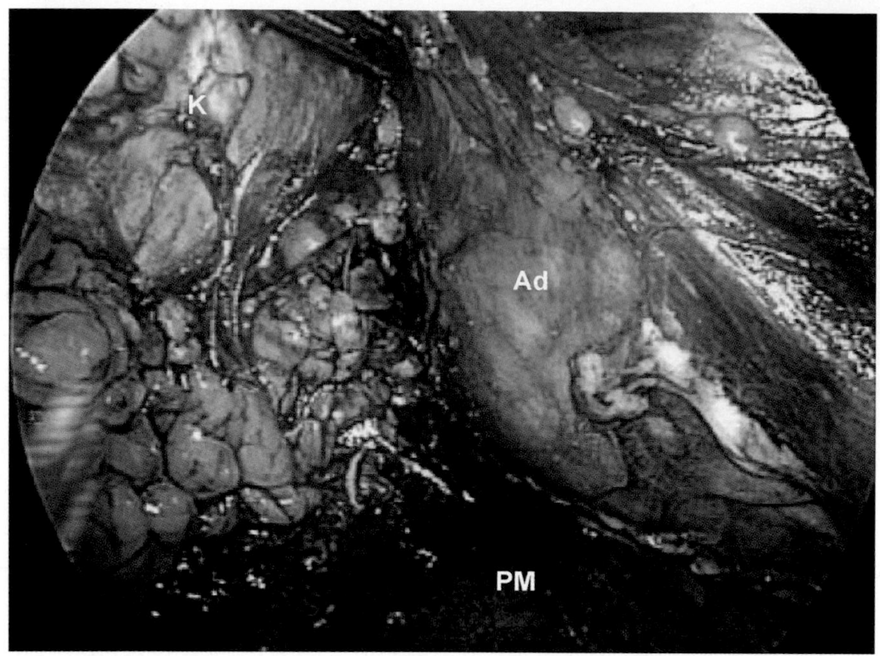

FIGURE 3.21. Retroperitoneoscopic left adrenalectomy. After the adrenal vein has been clipped and transected, the adrenal mass (Ad) is dissected off the upper pole of the kidney (K). PM = psoas muscle

The first 24 hours are critical to rule out any postoperative hemorrhage. As with all laparoscopic procedures, it is important for the healing process that the patient resumes walking on the evening of surgery. This facilitates resumption of bowel movements and helps reduce abdominal cramping. It also plays an important role in the prevention of deep venous phlebitis.

In the absence of complications, oral intake can be resumed on the morning after surgery.

The patient can be discharged on the evening of the day after surgery (unless this would be contraindicated by a specific medical reason related to the nature of the adrenal disease) after adequate pain control has been achieved with oral analgesics and oral intake of fluids has been resumed.

4 Radical Nephrectomy

Laparoscopic radical nephrectomy represents a watershed event in urologic oncology because it provided an alternative for removing a large solid organ using a minimally invasive approach. It continues to gain worldwide popularity and is becoming a standard procedure for the appropriate patient with an organ-confined T1 or T2 renal tumor. Depending on the individual patient characteristics, and particularly the training and expertise of the surgeon, either the transperitoneal or the retroperitoneal laparoscopic approach can be used. The retroperitoneal approach affords quicker access to the renal hilum and easier dissection in obese patients. However, it is a more difficult procedure to master, partly because the smaller working space makes entrapping the kidney more difficult, increasing the risk of conversion to open surgery. Urologists without a great deal of laparoscopic experience are advised to choose the transperitoneal approach.

Indications and Contraindications

In addition to the usual contraindications for laparoscopic surgery (uncorrected coagulopathy, cardiopulmonary instability, and abdominal sepsis), contraindications for laparoscopic radical nephrectomy also include inferior vena caval thrombus, bulky lymphadenopathy, and locally advanced disease that has invaded adjacent structures. Regardless, laparoscopic radical nephrectomy can be performed for most patients with organ-confined T1-T3a tumors, although collateral vessel and perirenal desmoplastic reaction can be significant if the tumor is large. However, large tumor size is only a relative contraindication, depending on the surgeon's experience and the characteristics of the individual tumor. Prior open surgery in the area increases the technical difficulty of the laparoscopic procedure, as does morbid obesity, although the retroperitoneal laparoscopic approach can be used successfully in these two situations.

Patient Preparation and Positioning

The following general instructions apply to patient preparation and positioning for both the transperitoneal and retroperitoneal approaches. Specific instructions relevant to each approach are included in the respective sections.

Anticoagulant medications must be discontinued well in advance of surgery. To prepare the bowels, the patient is instructed to ingest magnesium citrate during the afternoon before surgery. Broad-spectrum intravenous antibiotics are administered, and sequential compression stockings are applied preoperatively.

Patients are positioned on the operating table with their arms and legs maintained in a neutral position, and all dependent soft tissue and bony sites, including the head and neck, axilla, hip, knee, and ankle, are meticulously padded with egg-crate foam. The foam should then be reinforced to prevent postoperative neuromuscular strain.

Transperitoneal Technique

Patient Positioning and Port Placement

For the transperitoneal approach, the patient is positioned in a 60° flank position with the kidney bridge mildly elevated and the table mildly flexed. Pneumoperitoneum can be achieved just as safely using the Veress needle technique as during an open procedure.

After pneumoperitoneum has been established, the surgeon typically inserts 4 or 5 ports. A 10- or 12-mm primary trocar, maneuvered by the surgeon's left hand, is inserted at the lateral border of the rectus, at the level of the umbilicus; a 10- or 12-mm port 2-3 fingerbreadths lateral to the rectus muscle at the costal margin will be used by the surgeon's right hand. A third 10- or 12-mm port is inserted approximately 2-3 fingerbreadths below the costal margin at the lateral border of the rectus, and a 2-mm port is inserted near the costal margin at the anterior axillary line for lateral retraction of the kidney (Figure 4.1).

For right transperitoneal nephrectomy, a 5-mm port is inserted near the xiphoid for retraction of the liver.

For left transperitoneal nephrectomy, if needed for exposure, a 5-mm port is placed at the lateral border of the rectus, near the costal margin.

Mobilization of the Colon

Right Nephrectomy

During right nephrectomy, mobilization of the ascending colon is not essential. If necessary due to local constraints, such as adherences or fatty mesocolon, the line of Toldt is incised, and the

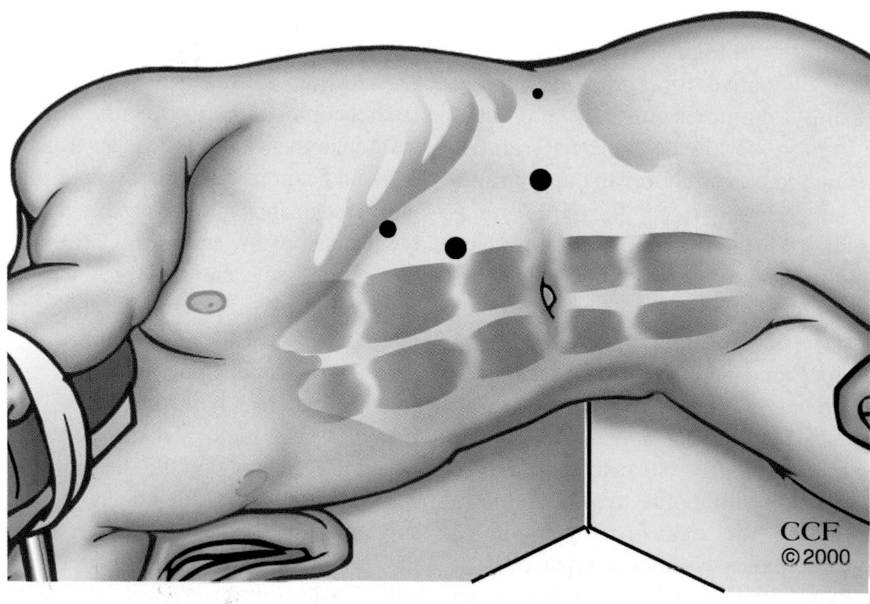

FIGURE 4.1. Transperitoneal left nephrectomy. The patient is positioned in a 60° flank position with the kidney bridge mildly elevated and the table mildly flexed. Four to five ports are necessary

colonic flexure reflected medially. This posterior peritoneotomy is extended transversely and medially along the inferior edge of the liver up to the vena cava. Kocher's maneuver is used to carefully mobilize the first two portions of the duodenum from the peritoneum medially until the anterior aspect of the inferior vena cava can be clearly seen (Figures 4.2 and 4.3).

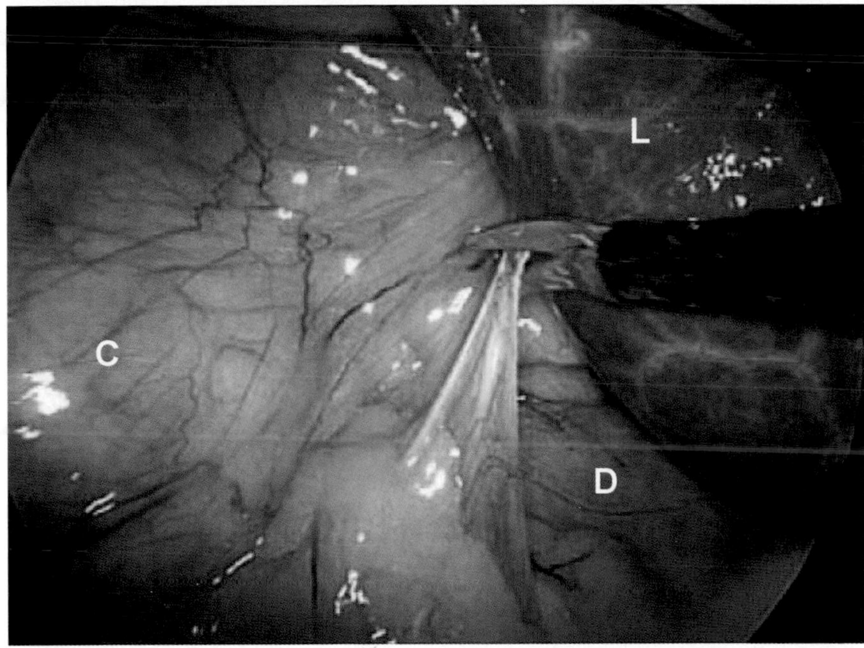

FIGURE 4.2. Transperitoneal right nephrectomy. Adhesions are released to free and lift the liver (L) and gain access to the duodenum (D), which will be mobilized to gain access to the inferior vena cava. C = colon

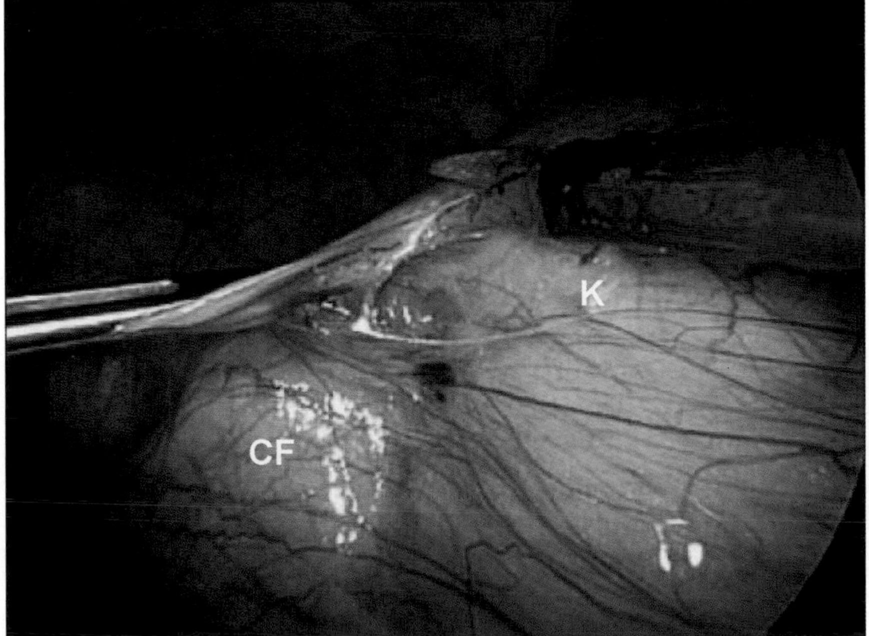

FIGURE 4.3. Transperitoneal right nephrectomy. The colonic flexure (CF) is dissected to free the inferior pole of the kidney (K). Extended dissection of the right colon is rarely necessary

Left Nephrectomy

During left nephrectomy, a formal mobilization of the descending colon is indispensable, as is the mobilization of the splenic flexure, spleen, and pancreas, because these structures almost completely cover the anterior aspect of Gerota's fascia. Thus, the splenocolic, splenorenal, and splenophrenic fascial attachments are released, allowing the spleen to be mobilized medially (Figures 4.4 and 4.5).

As in open surgery, the goal is to develop the correct avascular fascial plane between Gerota's fascia and the posterior aspect of the descending mesocolon.

Control of the Renal Vessels

A safe way to identify the renal hilum is to trace the gonadal vein toward the renal vein. This is done by identifying the ureter and gonadal vein, found below the lower pole of the kidney, lateral to the ipsilateral great vessels (aorta and vena cava). The psoas muscle can be visualized, and the ureter, gonadal vein, and adjacent fat can simply be followed to the hilum and the main hilar vessels (Figure 4.6). Taut anterolateral retraction on the divided ureter/gonadal vein stretches the renal hilum. Dissection along the psoas muscle and lateral border of the ipsilateral great vessels leads to the renal hilum. Anterolateral retraction of the lower pole of the kidney facilitates dissection of the posteriorly located renal artery, behind the renal vein (Figure 4.7).

Once the renal artery has been recognized and isolated, it is controlled with locking clips. However, a clip, even if locked, can fall off, particularly if the artery is transected too close to the clip, so applying 2 locking clips on the proximal section of the artery is recommended. After these clips have been applied, the artery can be transected a few millimeters away from the distal clip, leaving a stump that can help prevent the clip from falling off.

The renal vein is controlled with locking clips (using the same procedure as for the renal artery) or ligation, or if necessary, with a stapler (Figure 4.8). Any accessory renal hilar vessels should be controlled with locking clips.

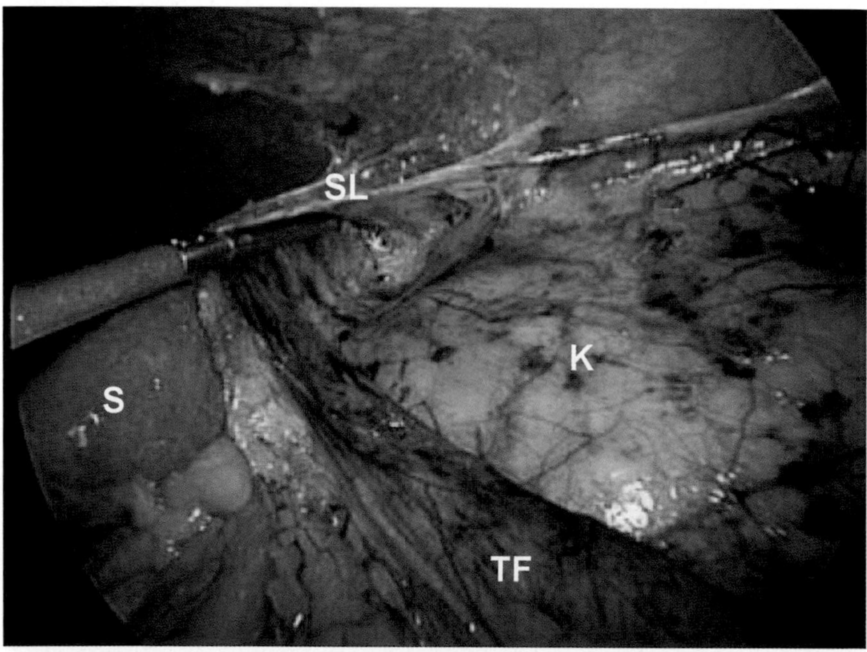

FIGURE 4.4. Transperitoneal left nephrectomy. The splenocolic ligaments (SL) are incised to allow the mobilization of the spleen (S) medially; Toldt's fascia (TF) should be incised extensively to expose Gerota's fascia and allow access to the left renal hilum. K = kidney

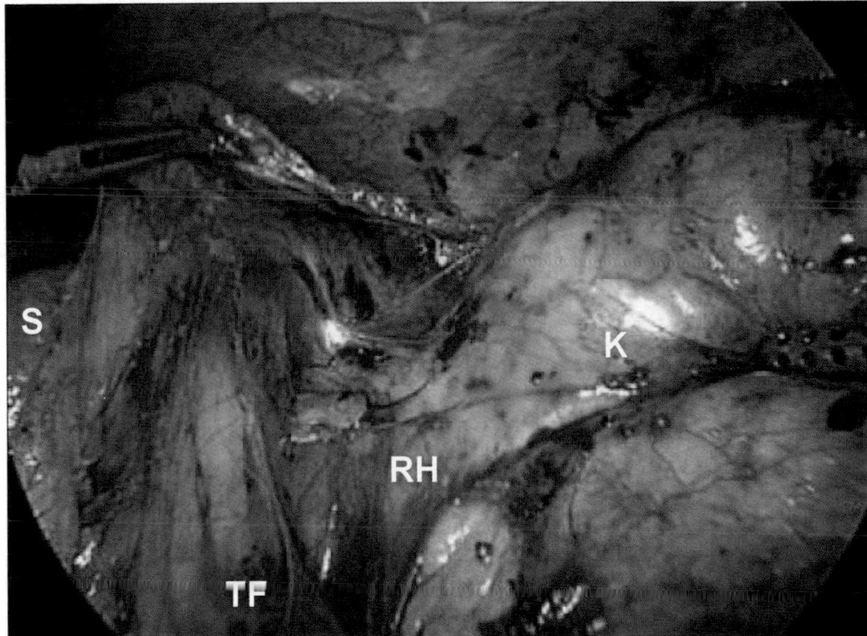

FIGURE 4.5. Transperitoneal left nephrectomy. Toldt's fascia (TF) is incised and the spleen (S) and descending colon are mobilized medially; the renal hilum (RH) becomes visible and should be incised extensively to expose Gerota's fascia and allow access to the left renal hilum. K = kidney

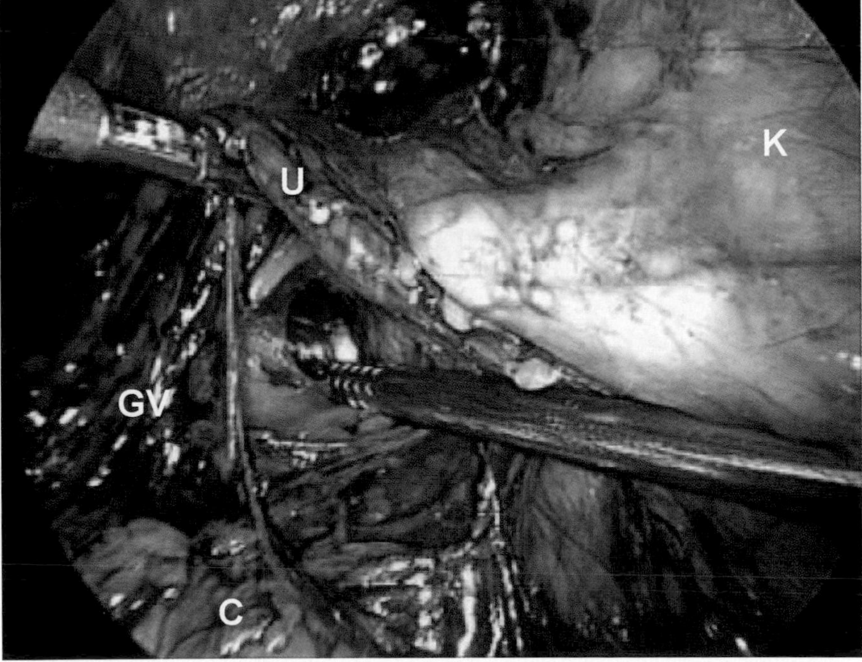

FIGURE 4.6. Laparoscopic right nephrectomy. The renal hilum can be found by identifying the ureter (U) and the gonadal vessel (GV) and tracing them upward to the main renal vessels. C = colon, K = kidney

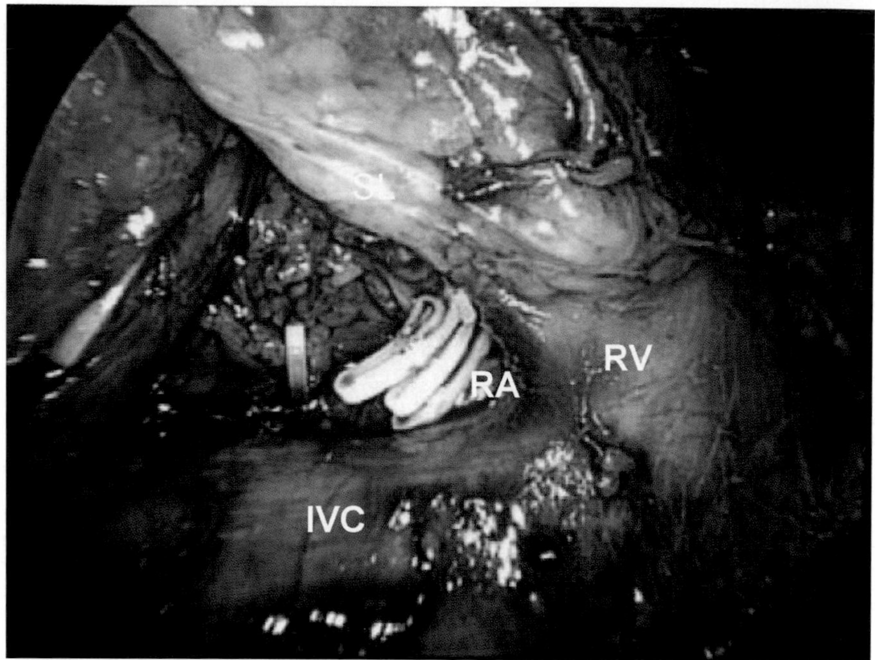

FIGURE 4.7. Laparoscopic left nephrectomy. Anterolateral retraction on the divided ureter/gonadal vein lifts the inferior renal pole and stretches the hilum, facilitating the dissection and ligation of the renal artery (RA) posterior to the renal vein (RV). IVC = inferior vena cava

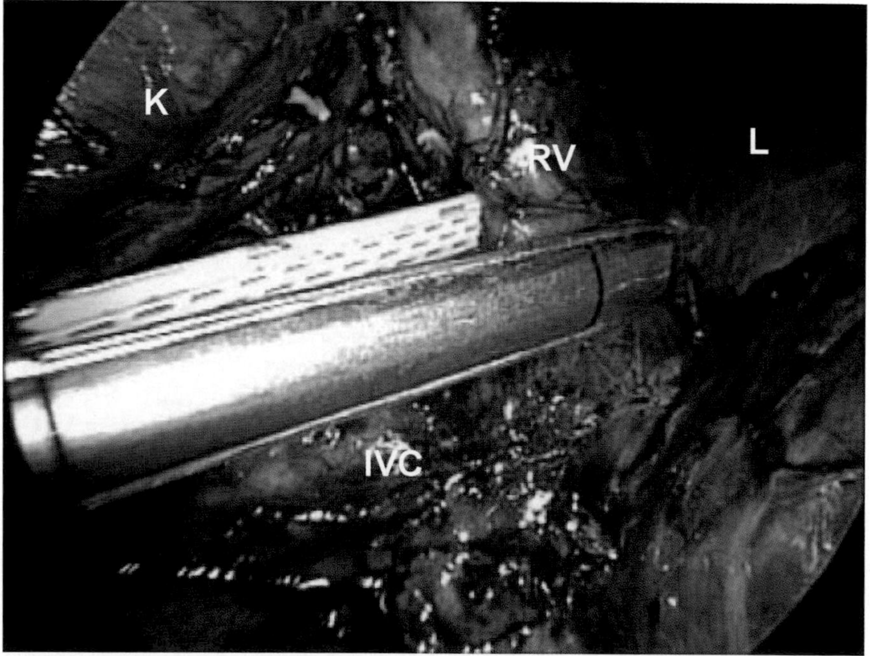

FIGURE 4.8. Laparoscopic left nephrectomy. The renal vein (RV) is controlled with a laparoscopic stapler or locking clips. Care should be taken to ensure that clips do not compromise the line of staple application. L = liver, K = kidney, IVC = inferior vena cava

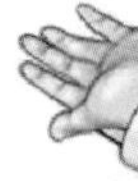

Bleeding from the Renal Hilum

Before detailed dissection of the renal vein and artery begins, the surgical field should be clear. In particular, all nearby vascular structures must be dissected with an appropriate extension to safely handle the bleeding. Use of monopolar cautery close to the renal vessels should be avoided, because this kind of electrocautery can easily result in unpredictable and major vascular damage.

Bleeding can initially be controlled with a peanut grasper. Lateral retraction of the kidney results in tension on the renal hilum, which usually slows the bleeding and facilitates the identification and inspection of the source. Once the source has been found, most renal hilar bleeding can be controlled by bipolar coagulation. If the bleeding is too severe for bipolar coagulation, clips can be used, but they must be applied directly to the source of the bleeding; an uncontrolled or blind use of clips is counterproductive and will compromise the potential use of sutures or a stapler. Indeed, if bleeding cannot be precisely controlled by use of stitches, it may be necessary to use a laparoscopic stapler over the whole hilum (vein and artery).

If the surgeon feels uncomfortable with a bleeding situation, there should not be any hesitation about converting to an open procedure (better sooner than later) to avoid unnecessary blood loss and subsequent circulatory complications.

Concomitant Adrenalectomy

Typically, concomitant adrenalectomy is recommended if any alteration in size, shape, or location of the adrenal gland has been found on preoperative CT scanning. Additionally, an upper pole or large tumor abutting the adrenal gland mandates adrenalectomy.

In concomitant adrenalectomy, the lateral surface of the ipsilateral great vessel is dissected bare, and all lymphatic fatty tissue in the area is excised; meanwhile, clips are placed on any lymphatic channels to avoid postoperative chylous ascites.

The main right adrenal vein is a thin-walled, short, stubby vessel directly entering the infrahepatic vena cava from the superomedial aspect of the right adrenal gland. Cephalad dissection along the vena cava allows identification of the adrenal vein, which is controlled with locking clips and then divided.

On the left side, the longer, narrower main left adrenal vein rises from the inferomedial aspect of the adrenal gland and drains directly into the left renal vein. It is similarly mobilized, clipped, and divided.

Specimen Entrapment

The specimen is entrapped in an endoscopy bag and can be extracted intact through a low suprapubic Pfannenstiel incision: the skin is incised at the level of the symphysis pubis, and the anterior rectus fascia is incised transversely somewhat higher up. This type of extraction incision is cosmetically preferred.

The abdomen is insufflated again to check for any remaining bleeding that needs to be controlled. Typically, no drain is placed.

Retroperitoneal Technique

Patient Positioning and Port Placement

Patient Positioning

The patient is secured in the standard 90° full-flank position. To maximize the space between the iliac crest and the lowermost rib, the kidney rest is elevated and the operating table flexed. However, to minimize neuromuscular strain, the kidney rest is lowered and the operating table unflexed once the laparoscopic tracers have been inserted and the location of the renal hilum identified. Thus, for most of the operation, the operating table remains straight, without any flexion.

Retroperitoneal Access

A 1.5-cm horizontal skin incision is made at the tip of the 12th rib. Two S retractors are used to separate the flank muscle fibers and to visualize the whitish thoracolumbar fascia; a 1-cm incision is created with the tip of an electrocautery blade. The surgeon inserts the tip of one index finger into the retroperitoneal space to perform a digital dissection along the anterior surface of the psoas muscle and fascia, staying outside Gerota's fascia. This creates a space for the balloon dilator (Figure 4.9).

Balloon Dissection

A balloon dilator is used to develop the retroperitoneal space. Six to eight pumps of a sphygmomanometer

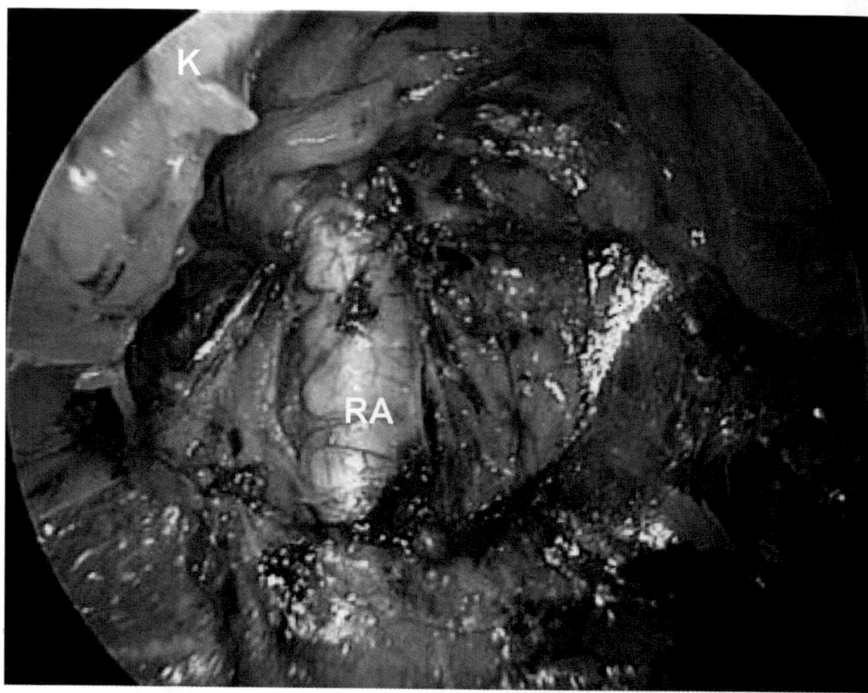

FIGURE 4.13. Retroperitoneoscopic left nephrectomy. After the kidney (K) has been retracted superiorly, the first landmark is the renal artery (RA), easily recognized by its forceful vertical pulsations

the TV monitor. Taut anterolateral retraction of the Gerota's fascia-covered kidney must be maintained constantly, using a 3-pronged metal retractor inserted through the anterior port and held in the surgeon's nondominant hand.

The electrocautery instrument is used to incise Gerota's fascia parallel, and 1-2 cm anterior, to the psoas muscle, directly in the region of the renal artery pulsations. The renal artery is circumferentially mobilized, clipped with 2 locking clips on the proximal side, and divided distally (Figure 4.14).

The renal vein, typically located anterior and caudal to the renal artery, is similarly mobilized and secured with locking clips, or if necessary, eventually a laparoscopic vascular stapler (Figure 4.15).

If a concomitant adrenalectomy is necessary, it is performed in a manner similar to the procedure used during a transperitoneal radical nephrectomy.

Lastly, the ureter and gonadal vein are identified, clipped, and divided (Figure 4.16).

Mobilization of the Kidney

The inferior renal pole is mobilized from the overlying peritoneum. Caudal traction on the partially mobilized kidney stretches the remaining perirenal attachments around the upper renal pole. The upper renal pole is mobilized from the inferior aspect of the adrenal gland (in adrenal-sparing nephrectomy) or from the inferior surface of the diaphragm (if concomitant adrenalectomy is performed). Electrocautery should not be used along the undersurface of the peritoneal envelope, to guard against thermal injury to intra-abdominal viscera, including the bowel. Indeed, although bowel loops are out of sight, they must never be out of mind, because they are separated from the surgical field by only the thin peritoneum, with potential for unrecognized transmural injury.

Specimen Entrapment

The specimen is entrapped in an endoscopy bag. The intact extraction can be performed through

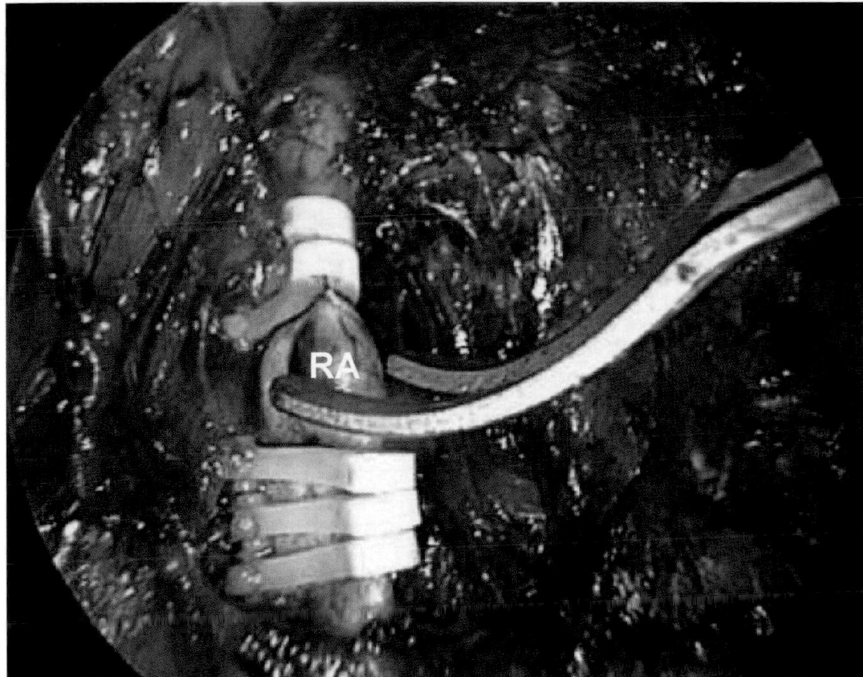

FIGURE 4.14. Retroperitoneoscopic left nephrectomy. The renal artery (RA) is circumferentially dissected and then ligated with locking clips

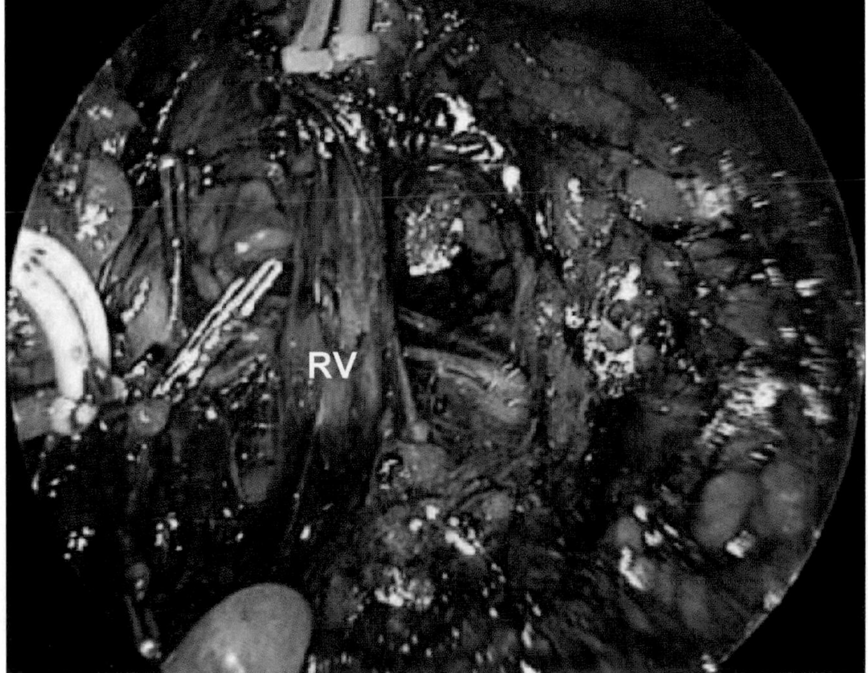

FIGURE 4.15. Retroperitoneoscopic left nephrectomy. The renal vein (RV) is located anterior and caudal to the renal artery. It often appears flattened after the renal artery has been ligated, and it can easily be secured with locking clips

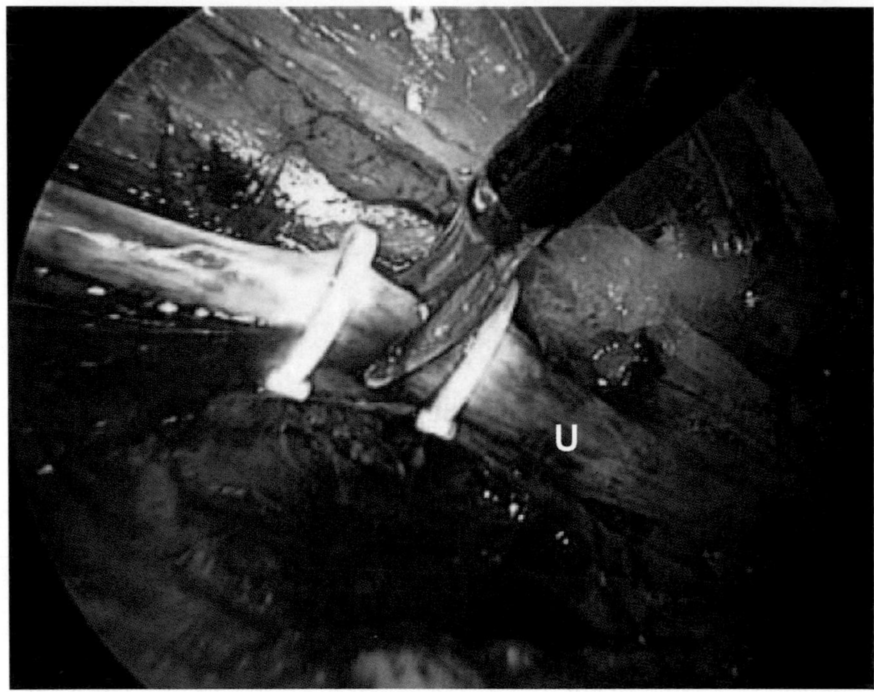

FIGURE 4.16. Retroperitoneoscopic left nephrectomy. The ureter (U) is identified and transected between two clips

a Pfannenstiel incision, while staying completely extraperitoneal. Typically, no drain is placed.

Renal Vein Thrombus

Laparoscopic radical nephrectomy has been used for renal cell carcinoma associated with level 1 renal vein thrombus.

Intraoperative flexible ultrasonography can be used to precisely confirm the proximal extent of the renal vein tumor thrombus. Thus, the surgeon can assess the technical feasibility of complete laparoscopic excision with negative vascular margins. Initially, the main renal artery is occluded by clipping, then the renal vein is mobilized. The proximal, thrombus-free segment of the renal vein usually appears flat because it is devoid of blood flow; this can be clearly differentiated from the distended, thrombus-bearing distal renal vein. Although, typically, this distinction is clearly visible laparoscopically, it can be further confirmed by laparoscopic contact ultrasonography. Using locking clips or a laparoscopic stapler, the renal vein is secured proximal (medial) to the thrombus.

After the specimen has been entrapped and extracted, retroperitoneal lymph node dissection should be considered, especially in large lesions when the risk of regional lymphadenopathy is increased. The development of new medications with significant efficacy in metastatic renal cell carcinoma may justify the more thorough retroperitoneal lymph node dissection in these situations.

Postoperative Care

The patient should begin walking on the evening of surgery. Two laxative suppositories can be administered on the morning after surgery, and oral intake can be resumed.

In more than 70% of cases, the patient can be discharged on the evening of the day after surgery, after adequate pain control has been achieved with oral analgesics, and oral intake of fluids has been resumed.

5
Partial Nephrectomy

Small, incidental renal tumors are being diagnosed with increasing frequency as a result of improved imaging technologies. In these cases, radical nephrectomy is not the surgery of choice. Partial nephrectomy affords long-term oncologic outcomes similar to those in radical nephrectomy with the benefit of preserving and maintaining a high glomerular filtration rate. Laparoscopic partial nephrectomy is an accepted minimally invasive nephron-sparing alternative for selected renal masses. As more surgeons develop the necessary confidence and expertise in laparoscopic surgery, the number of complex reconstructive and oncologic procedures performed laparoscopically will likely rise.

This chapter describes one technique for laparoscopic partial nephrectomy, including its indications and contraindications, the necessary instrumentation, and technical tips and nuances. In general, this technique is applicable to either the transperitoneal or retroperitoneal approach, with any surgical differences noted accordingly.

Indications and Contraindications

Laparoscopic partial nephrectomy was once reserved for small, superficial, peripheral, exophytic renal masses, for which the technically straightforward wedge resection was sufficient. Increasing experience has allowed the indications of laparoscopic partial nephrectomy to be expanded to include more complex cases in which nephron preservation is imperative: deeply infiltrating central tumors requiring intentional pelvicaliceal entry and repair, large tumors requiring heminephrectomy (resection of at least 30% of the kidney), hilar tumors, and tumors in a solitary kidney—which necessitated the development of laparoscopic techniques for renal hypothermia.

Because laparoscopic partial nephrectomy is a technically demanding, advanced minimally invasive procedure, the surgeon must have considerable laparoscopic experience and expertise.

Hilar Dissection

First the renal hilum is dissected, then the kidney is mobilized, and finally the tumor is approached.

On the right side, the liver is retracted anteriorly; on the left side, the spleen and pancreas are reflected medially. The ipsilateral colon is mobilized on either side, but more so on the left than on the right. The ureter and gonadal vein packet is dissected en bloc and lifted anteriorly off the psoas muscle.

Dissection is carried toward the renal vein, which is mobilized enough that the surgeon can appreciate its precise location and visualize the anterior surface in its entirety. The renal vein and artery are not individually skeletonized during laparoscopic partial nephrectomy, for a number of reasons: doing so can induce renal artery vasospasm or risk iatrogenic vascular injury, it is often unnecessary to achieve adequate clamping, and it takes approximately 30 minutes of important operating time that could be spent on the primary purpose of the procedure.

Superior to the renal hilum, the adrenal gland is dissected off the medial aspect of the upper pole kidney, which is then mobilized anteriorly off the psoas muscle. Essentially, the anterior, posterior, inferior, and superior aspects of the en bloc renal hilum, with some hilar fat intact, are prepared (Figure 5.1). These maneuvers allow the Satinsky vascular clamp to be deployed across the en bloc renal hilum with safety and confidence. Care must be taken not to miss any secondary renal arteries or veins.

Alternatively, individual bulldog clamps can be placed on the renal artery and vein separately, after each vascular structure has been circumferentially mobilized.

Mobilization of the Kidney

Gerota's fascia is entered and the fat removed from most of the renal surface. This defatting is advised for a number of reasons: the kidney becomes more

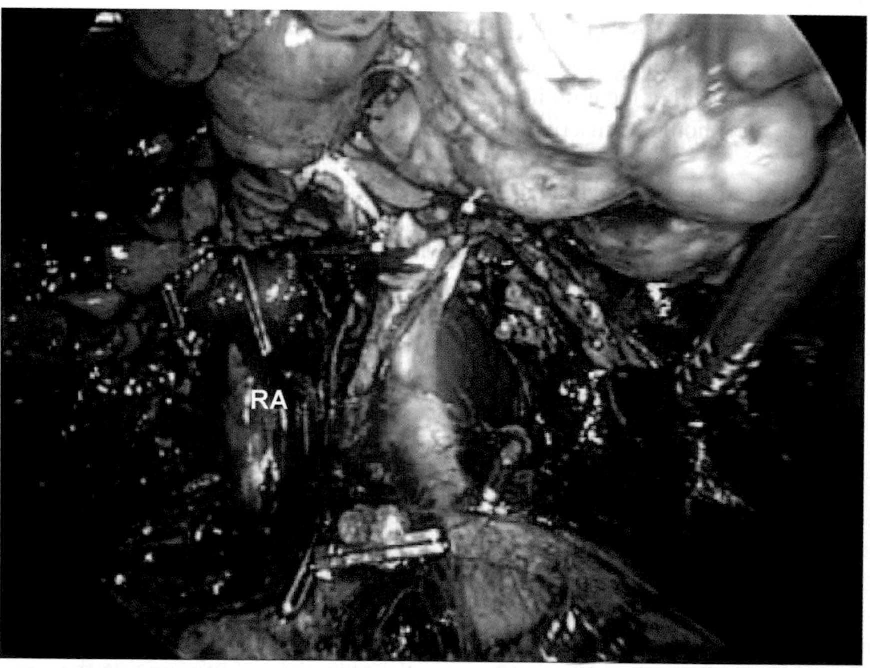

FIGURE 5.1. Right retroperitoneoscopic partial nephrectomy. The renal hilum is dissected en bloc, and no attempt is made to individualize the vein and artery. The ureter should be kept out of the clamping area. RA = renal artery

mobile, the surgeon is more likely to visualize secondary satellite tumors, and it allows multidirectional intraoperative ultrasound viewing and therefore more versatility for tumor resection and suturing angles.

However, the perirenal fat overlying the tumor and its vicinity should be maintained intact, thereby allowing adequate staging of potential T3a tumors, and eventually serving, with caution, as a handle during tumor resection.

Intraoperative Ultrasonography

Thorough real-time ultrasonographic examination of the tumor is essential. A steerable, flexible, color Doppler ultrasound probe with a 10-mm shaft is used to facilitate planning of tumor resection. Information is obtained regarding tumor size, invasion depth, distance of tumor from pelvicaliceal system, and identification of any large peritumoral blood vessels. Additionally, a search can be made for any small satellite tumors that may have been missed on preoperative CT scanning (Figure 5.2).

Using real-time ultrasonographic guidance, the surgeon can propose a line of excision by circumferentially scoring around the tumor with the tip of a monopolar electrocautery probe. The oncologic adequacy of this scored margin is reconfirmed ultrasonographically before initiating tumor resection.

Hilar Clamping

A bloodless field is essential for a technically precise excision and extraction of the tumor, as well as for parenchymal repair. This ideal surgical field is best achieved with hilar clamping. As mentioned above, clamping the hilum en bloc is a safe option, but the entire renal hilum must be enclosed within the jaws of the Satinsky clamp: the clamp is fully opened and slowly advanced over the renal hilum in a deliberate manner, such that the jaw of the clamp facing the surgeon is anterior to the renal vein, while the posterior jaw hugs the psoas muscle. This reliably includes the renal artery and renal vein within the clamp jaws, along with some hilar fat that serves to cushion the renal vessels against clamp injury. The Satinsky clamp must be placed on the hilum medial enough to the ureter and renal pelvis to avoid ureteral crush injury (Figure 5.3).

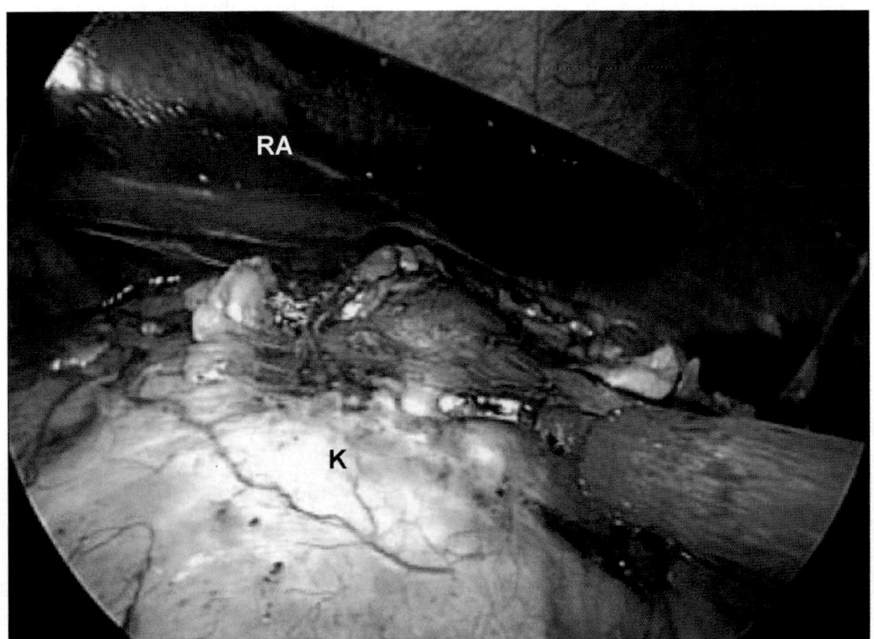

FIGURE 5.2. Right laparoscopic partial nephrectomy. Intraoperative ultrasonography is essential for obtaining information regarding tumor size, invasion depth, distance of tumor from pelvicaliceal system, identification of any large peritumoral blood vessels, and any small satellite tumors that may not have been visible on preoperative CT scanning

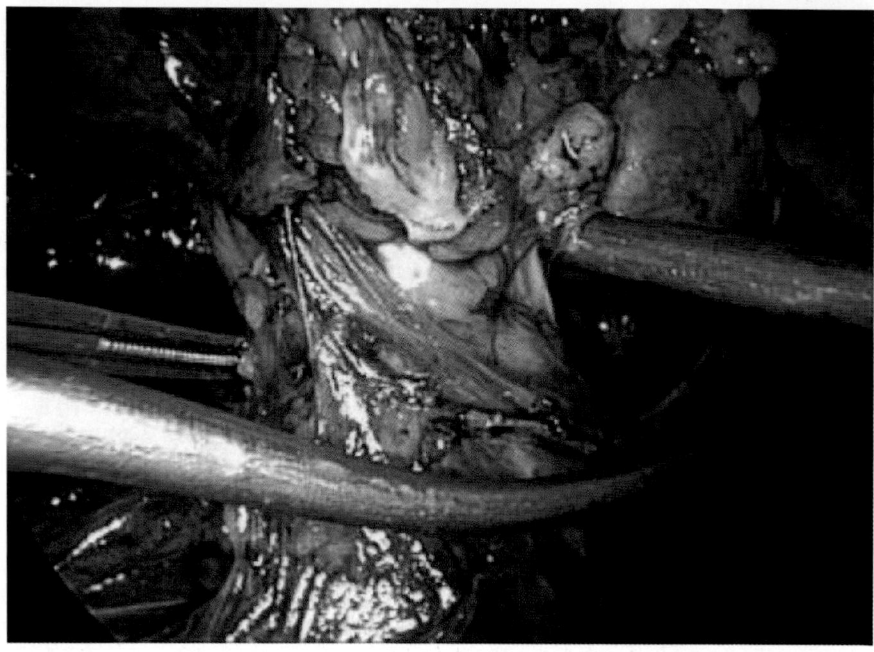

FIGURE 5.3. Right laparoscopic partial nephrectomy. The renal hilum is dissected en bloc, and a laparoscopic Satinsky clamp is applied. The ureter has been dissected to prevent it from being clamped

During the retroperitoneal approach, the jaw of the clamp facing the surgeon lies posterior to the renal artery, while the jaw of the other clamp must be anatomically anterior enough to safely encompass the renal vein. Additionally, the renal hilar structures must be separated from the peritoneum so that the clamp cannot accidentally enter the peritoneum.

The anesthesiologist starts a time clock to monitor the duration of warm ischemia.

Tumor Resection

Once the hilum is clamped, tumor resection is initiated. The renal capsule is circumferentially incised with electrocautery (Figure 5.4). Tumor resection is then performed using cold shears. Nondisposable scissors are the best because they are more rigid and therefore more stable, and their jaws are larger than those of disposable endoshears. Depth of tumor resection is guided by the information obtained from the preoperative CT scan, the intraoperative ultrasound examination, and laparoscopic visual clues during resection (Figures 5.5 to 5.7).

The aim is to obtain a margin of at least 0.5 cm around the tumor. To a less experienced surgeon, this margin may visually appear as though an excessive amount of kidney is being excised. However, the magnification of the laparoscope must be remembered. After the tumor has been extracted, inspecting the specimen along with the pathologist is an invaluable learning experience for the surgeon.

Pelvicaliceal Repair and Parenchymal Hemostasis

The bed of the partial nephrectomy defect is oversewn with a running 2-0 Vicryl suture on a CT-1 needle. This suturing has two specific goals: watertight repair of any pelvicaliceal system entry confirmed by retrograde injection of dilute indigo carmine through the ureteral catheter; and oversewing of any large transected intrarenal blood vessels, the majority of which lie in the vicinity of the renal sinus. Individual suture repair with figure-8 stitches can be performed on any additional blood vessels as necessary (Figures 5.8 and 5.9).

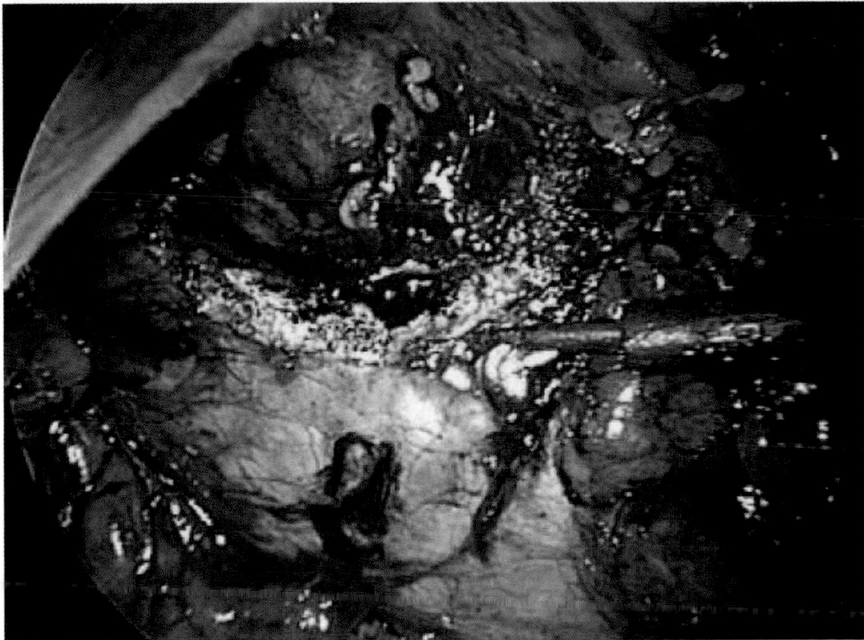

FIGURE 5.4. Right retroperitoneoscopic partial nephrectomy. After the hilum has been clamped, the renal capsule is circumferentially incised to mark the resection line

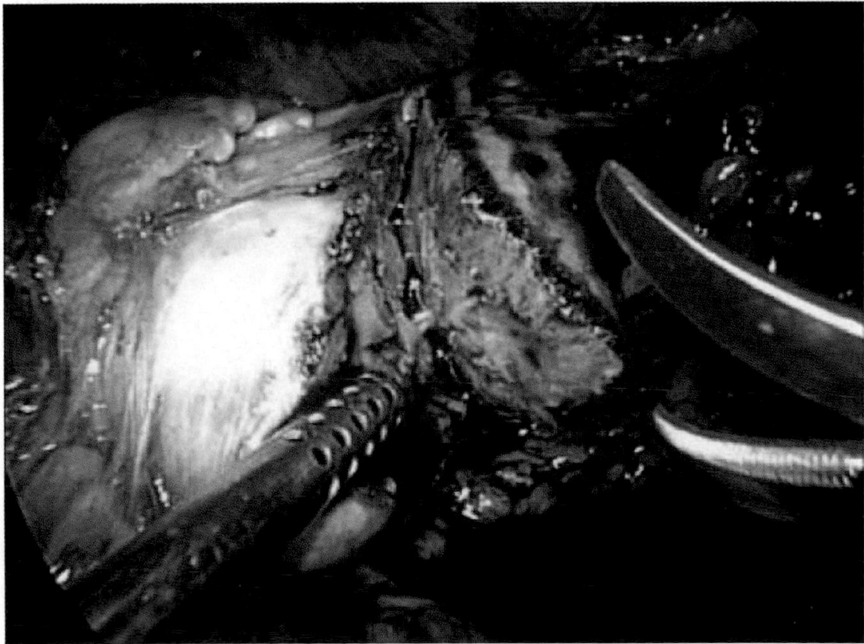

FIGURE 5.5. Right laparoscopic partial nephrectomy. The renal parenchyma is resectioned using cold shears, to avoid smoke and keep the resection line clear so that any structures needing repair can be seen. Dissection too close to the tumor can adversely affect the parenchymal resectioning

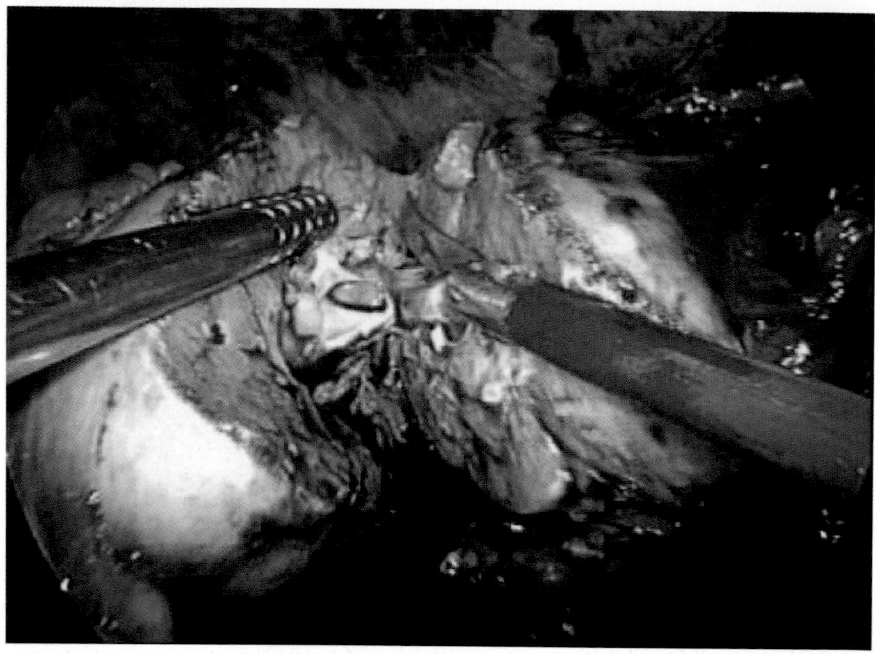

FIGURE 5.6. Right laparoscopic partial nephrectomy. A suction device to aspirate bleeding is essential during parenchymal resection

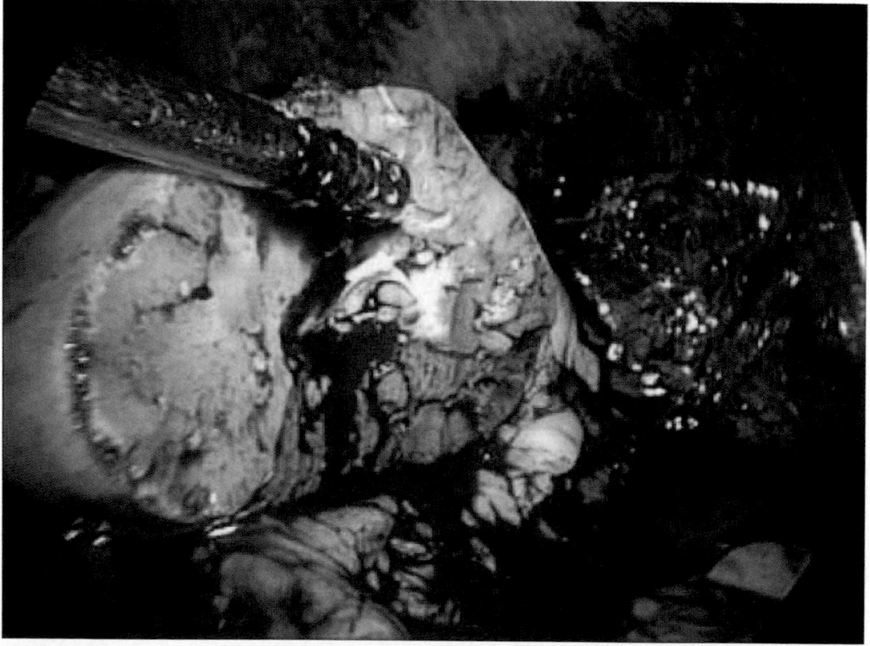

FIGURE 5.7. Right laparoscopic partial nephrectomy. After the tumor has been resected, the area is carefully examined to ensure there is no residual tumor in the bed site and to identify the caliceal opening and location of vessels

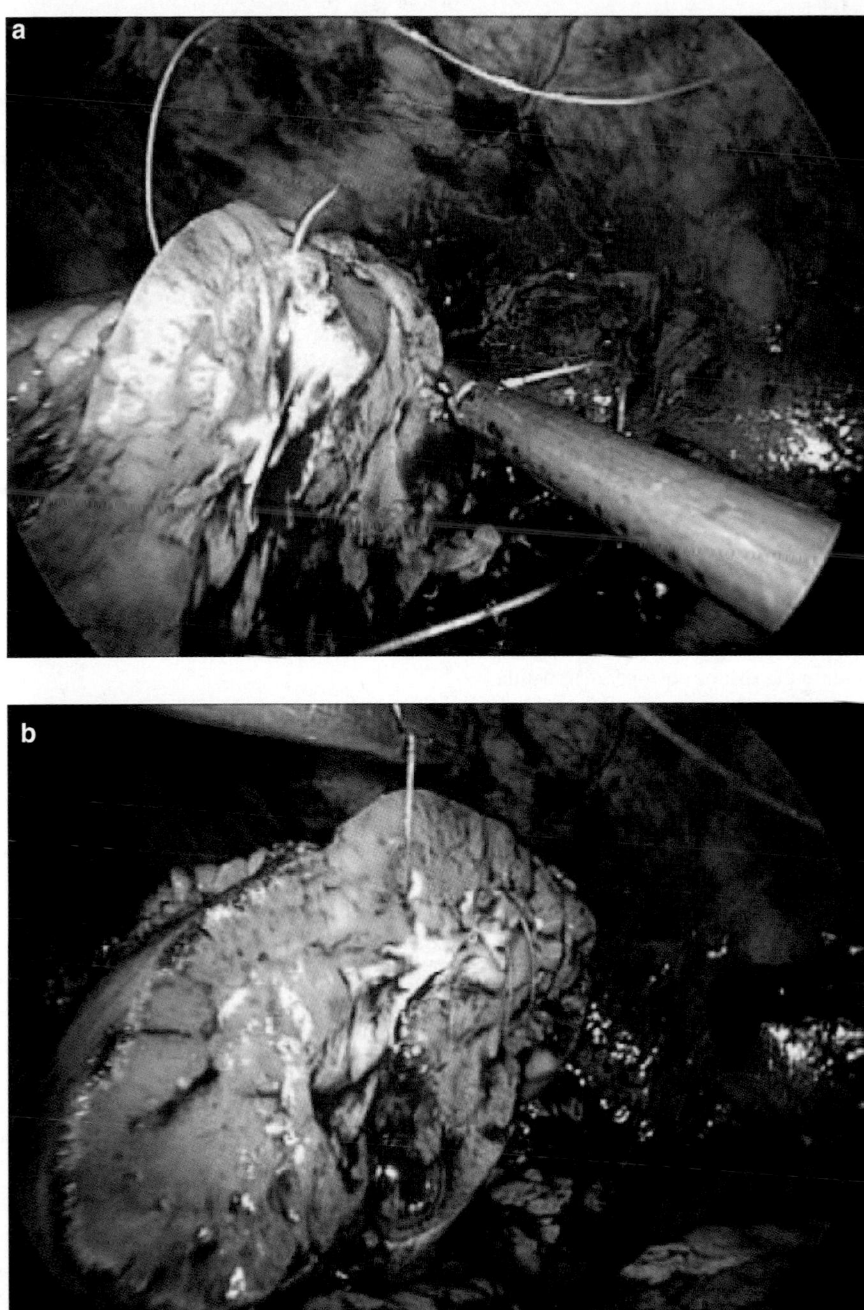

FIGURE 5.8. **(a)** Right laparoscopic partial nephrectomy. The bed of the partial nephrectomy is oversewn with a running suture using 2-0 Vicryl on a CT-1 needle to achieve a precise watertight repair and hemostasis. **(b)** Right laparoscopic partial nephrectomy. The bed of the partial nephrectomy is oversewn with a running suture using 2-0 Vicryl on a CT-1 needle to achieve a precise watertight repair and hemostasis

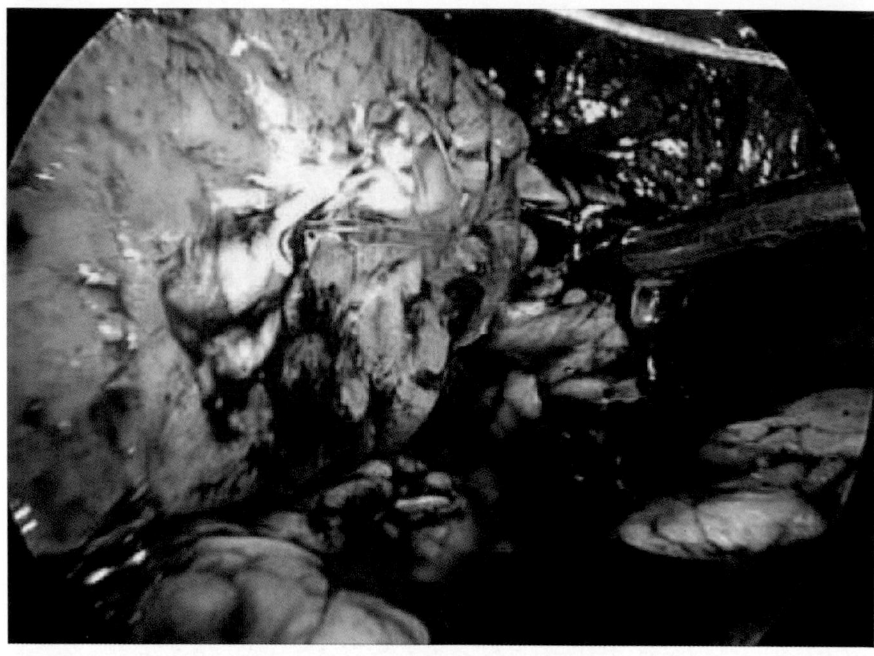

FIGURE 5.9. Right laparoscopic partial nephrectomy. Incomplete closure of a caliceal defect will be exposed by retrograde injection of dilute indigo carmine through the ureteral catheter. A figure-8 or U-stitch will create a watertight closure and decrease the risk of postoperative fistula

Parenchymal renorrhaphy is performed with 1 Vicryl on a CTX needle. The suture is cut to port length, and a locking clip is preplaced 4-5 cm from the tail end of the suture to serve as a pledget. Renal parenchymal stitches are placed over a preprepared oxidized cellulose bolster. These parenchymal stitches require meticulous execution, with the desired angle and depth of needle passage preplanned to prevent multiple passages, thus minimizing possible puncture injury to the intrarenal blood vessels. This prefashioned bolster is positioned underneath the suture loop. The 5-mm metal applicator is used to apply a gelatin matrix thrombin sealant directly onto the partial nephrectomy bed underneath the bolster. The suture is tightened, compressing the bolster firmly onto the partial nephrectomy bed. Another locking clip is placed on the exiting suture flush with the parenchyma, thus maintaining consistent pressure. The two suture tails are tied together with a surgeon's knot. With the suture cinched down, an assistant grasps the knot with a Maryland grasper to hold the suture secure at this point of maximal tension. The surgeon places two additional knots, securing the stitch.

Merely placing a clip as a pledget on either end of the suture does not provide enough security of parenchymal compression, leaving the potential for bleeding from the edges of the partial nephrectomy defect. As such, tying the suture tails across the bolster over the partial nephrectomy is important to coapt the edges of the parenchymal defect (Figures 5.10 and 5.11).

Typically, between 3 and 5 parenchymal renorrhaphy sutures are required to close the entire defect.

Hilar Unclamping and Specimen Entrapment

A repeat 12.5-gm dose of mannitol and 10-20 mg of furosemide are administered intravenously 1-2 minutes before unclamping the renal hilum.

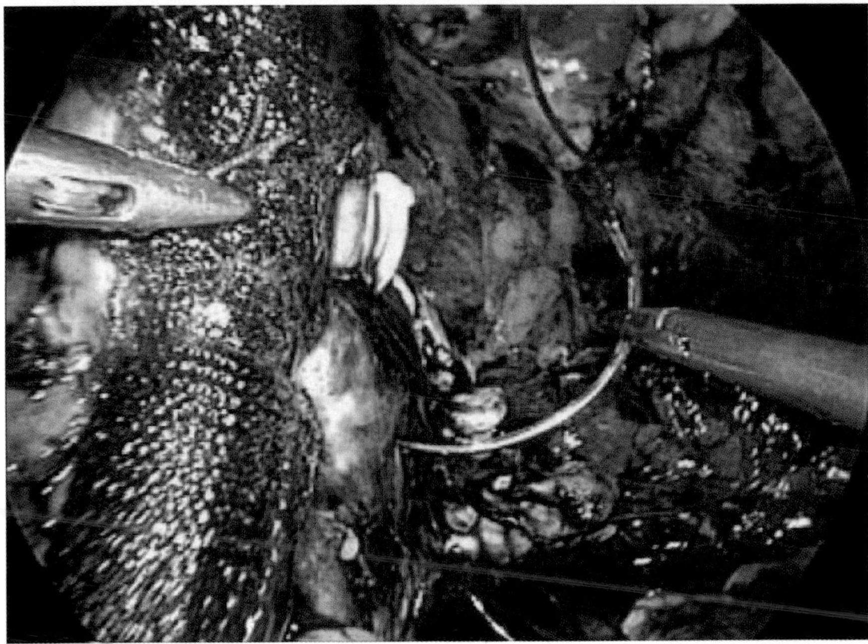

FIGURE 5.10. Right laparoscopic partial nephrectomy. Parenchymal renorrhaphy is performed with 1-0 Vicryl on a CTX needle, run over a prefashioned bolster positioned under the suture loops

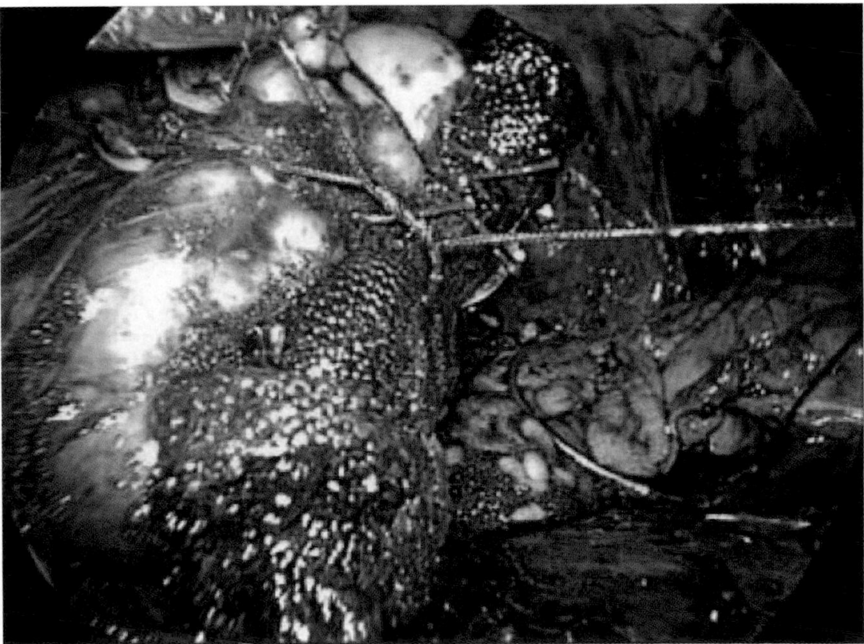

FIGURE 5.11. Right laparoscopic partial nephrectomy. A gelatin thrombin sealant is layered directly onto the bed of the resection; then the suture tails are ligated over the bolster to coapt the parenchymal edges

The Satinsky clamp jaws are opened, but not yet removed, to assess the adequacy of hemostasis from the partial nephrectomy bed. Once the surgeon is satisfied with hemostasis, the clamp (or bulldogs, if they were used) is slowly and carefully removed, first from the vein and then from the artery, under direct visualization.

The entrapped specimen is extracted intact (Figure 5.12) by slightly extending one of the port-site incisions.

A Jackson-Pratt drain is placed during transperitoneal laparoscopic partial nephrectomy, and a Penrose drain is placed after a retroperitoneal laparoscopic partial nephrectomy. The fascia at the 10- or 12-mm port sites is closed with a Carter-Thompson needle. The partial nephrectomy bed is reinspected laparoscopically after 5-10 minutes of desufflation to confirm complete hemostasis.

Renal Hypothermia

When necessary, renal hypothermia can be achieved by any of three different methods. Retrograde ureteral perfusion via the ureteric catheter that is inserted before the laparoscopic procedure begins has been used for many years. Intra-arterial perfusion via percutaneous catheterization of the femoral artery has been done more recently.

A technique using ice-slush to induce hypothermia has also been developed for laparoscopic partial nephrectomy. Finely crushed ice slurry is preloaded into 30-mL syringes, the nozzle ends of which have been cut off. The mobilized kidney is entrapped in an endoscopy bag, and the drawstring cinched down around the intact renal hilum to completely entrap the kidney. The renal hilum is clamped with a Satinsky clamp. The bottom end of the bag is retrieved outside the abdomen through the inferior pararectal port site. The bottom end is opened, and the preloaded syringes rapidly fill the intra-abdominal bag with ice slurry. Typically, 4-7 minutes are required to fill the bag with 600-900 mL of ice slurry, thus surrounding the entire kidney under laparoscopic visualization. After allowing 10 minutes to achieve core renal cooling, the bag is incised, the ice crystals removed from the vicinity of the tumor, and partial nephrectomy completed.

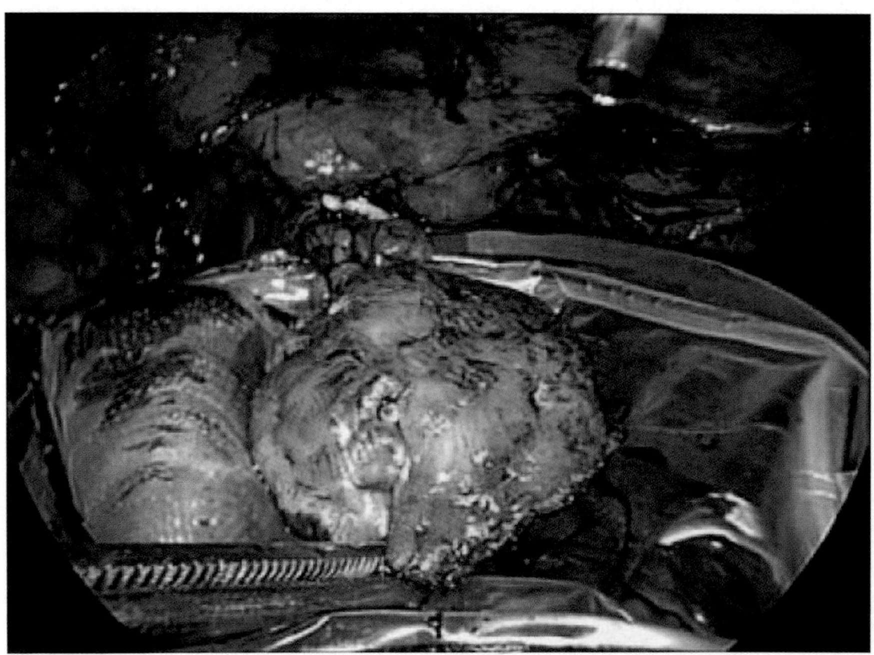

FIGURE 5.12. Right retroperitoneoscopic partial nephrectomy. The risk of tumor seeding is minimized by immediately placing the newly freed specimen in a laparoscopic bag

Complications

Some type of complication occurs in about one-third of patients. Most are urological but others include hemorrhage and urine leak. Conversion to open partial nephrectomy is rarely needed but is always a possible complication.

The more common use of hemostatic agents such as gelatin matrix thrombin sealant, which is routinely used during laparoscopic partial nephrectomy, has decreased the rate of complications.

Postoperative Care

Strict bed rest is advised for 24 hours after surgery, followed by a gradual return to mobility.

The ureteral and Foley catheters are removed 2 days after surgery as the patient begins ambulation. The perirenal drain is maintained for at least 3-5 days and removed when the drainage is less than 50 mL/day for 3 consecutive days.

After discharge from the hospital, restricted activity is advised for 2 weeks. Any physical activity that can potentially jar the renal remnant is inadvisable during the early postoperative period.

A MAG-3 radionuclide scan is performed 4 weeks after surgery to evaluate renal function and to assess the integrity of the pelvicaliceal system.

6
Nephroureterectomy

Tumor stage and grade are the major predictors of recurrence and survival in upper urinary tract transitional cell carcinoma. If the disease is papillary and/or low grade, an endourological approach (retrograde or antegrade) is a minimally invasive surgical alternative, particular in patients with problematic kidney function or bilateral disease. Invasive and/or high-grade tumors are associated with a high recurrence rate and poorer prognosis, and radical nephroureterectomy remains the treatment of choice. While highly efficacious for disease control, conventional nephroureterectomy requires two incisions or one long midline incision and results in significant morbidity with pain and extended convalescence. With advances in laparoscopic surgery, laparoscopic nephroureterectomy has minimized morbidity and become a viable alternative to conventional nephroureterectomy.

Patient Preparation

Bowel preparation is generally limited to clear liquid diet for the day before surgery, and a laxative suppository the night before surgery.

A first-generation cephalosporin is administered when anesthesia is introduced.

In obese patients or in patients with a history of deep venous thrombosis, 5,000 IU of heparin should be given subcutaneously and continued postoperatively until the patient is ambulatory.

Operating Room Preparation

Instruments

The personal preferences of the surgeon should determine the specific instruments chosen for the procedure. The instrument set for nephroureterectomy is similar to that for radical nephrectomy.

Patient Positioning

First, general endotracheal anesthesia is induced, and the patient's stomach decompressed with an orogastric tube.

The upper body is placed in a full flank position with the affected kidney on top, while the pelvis is somewhat rotated toward a supine position.

Orthopedic table braces to support the patient's shoulder and hip help maintain the proper position. The operating table is flexed according to the patient's flexibility and the surgeon's preference. The table should be straightened during surgery when it no longer improves exposure.

All bony prominences must be padded. The arm opposite the affected kidney is padded, and the axillary area carefully positioned. The ipsilateral arm is placed on an arm-board. Finally, the patient is secured on the table with one strap over the chest and one over the hip for additional safety, particularly when rotating the table (Figure 6.1).

A Foley catheter is introduced after the patient has been draped, providing sterile access to the catheter during surgery.

Surgical Team

A standard organization of all lines and cords, preferably with all approaching the operating table from one direction, makes the operation easier. Because visibility of the intraoperative picture is crucial for the surgeon and the assistant, two monitors must be available, placed on each side at the patient's shoulder level.

The surgeon and the camera assistant are positioned opposite the affected kidney, while the surgical assistant and scrub nurse are positioned on the ipsilateral side. Important tools, such as the insufflator, camera, light source, and electrocautery device, must be positioned across from the surgeon for direct control.

Operative Technique

Transperitoneal, extraperitoneal, and hand-assisted approaches have been described for laparoscopic nephroureterectomy. Various rationales have been used to support both transperitoneal and retroperitoneal techniques. In general, laparoscopic nephroureterectomy is feasible with acceptable morbidity and overall favorable perioperative outcomes regardless of the specific laparoscopic approach used. The transperitoneal technique is described below, based on the authors' preference.

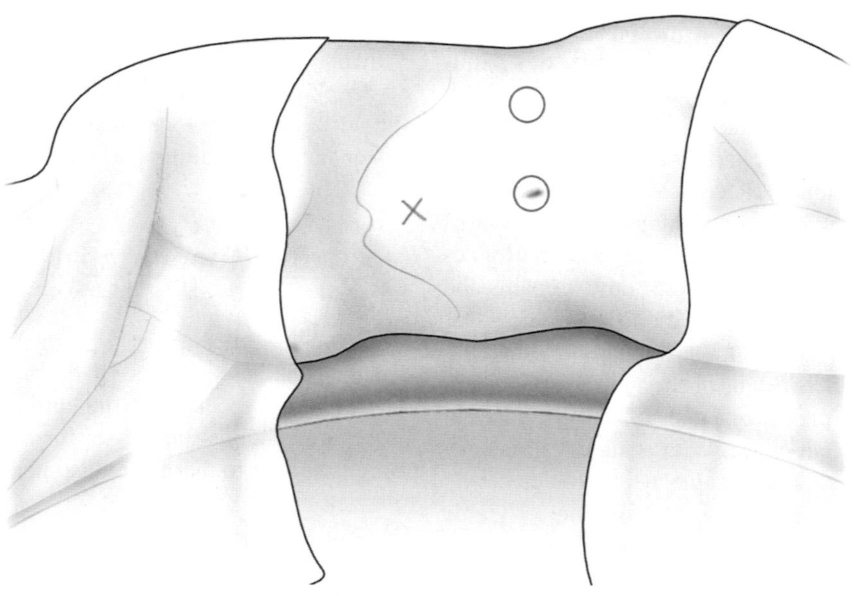

FIGURE 6.1. Position of the patient for left laparoscopic nephroureterectomy. The upper body is in a flank position, while the pelvis is slightly rotated toward a supine position, allowing easier access to the lower portion of the ureter. The placement of the main ports is noted. The Gibson incision should be drawn on the skin with a surgical pen while the patient is in a supine position, before the skin is prepared

Transperitoneal Access and Port Placement

After a periumbilical incision has been made, a Veress needle is introduced into the peritoneal cavity and a pneumoperitoneum obtained (15 to 20 mmHg). Alternatively, the pneumoperitoneum can be obtained by performing a mini-laparotomy with introduction of a Hasson trocar. A 10/12-mm trocar for optical access is placed at the periumbilical site, and the abdominal pressure set at 15 mmHg. In moderately and severely obese patients, the camera port must be placed more laterally in the pararectal area, at the level of the umbilicus. A 0° laparoscope is inserted, and the peritoneal cavity inspected for any potential injury.

Under direct visual control, two additional trocars are placed. One 5-mm trocar is placed 2 cm below the costal margin in the midclavicular line. A second trocar (10/12-mm), is placed in the pararectal area just distal of the umbilicus. After mobilization of the colon, a fourth trocar, 5-mm, is usually placed in the flank area, subcostal in the axillary line (Figure 6.2).

To facilitate visualization of the retroperitoneum behind the colon, the surgeon may also use a 30° laparoscope.

Control of the Renal Vessels and Mobilization of the Kidney

The dissection of the kidney follows the same steps as in radical nephrectomy. The line of Toldt is incised, and the colon completely mobilized away from the kidney. As in radical nephrectomy, staying in the exact plane between the colon and the retroperitoneum will avoid "getting lost" in the retroperitoneal fatty tissue and will keep the kidney attached to the abdominal sidewall, facilitating hilar dissection later in the procedure.

In contrast to radical nephrectomy, complete mobilization of the entire colon (either ascending or descending) from the colonic flexure (left as well as right) to the pelvis is mandatory: anatomic dissection with wide exposure of all the important structures, particular the vascular structures, is key to a safe and successful procedure.

Right Nephroureterectomy

The liver is retracted with a grasper introduced over an additional 5-mm trocar placed in the midline approximately 2 cm below the xiphoid. The liver is raised with the grasper and fixed to tissue on the right abdominal wall.

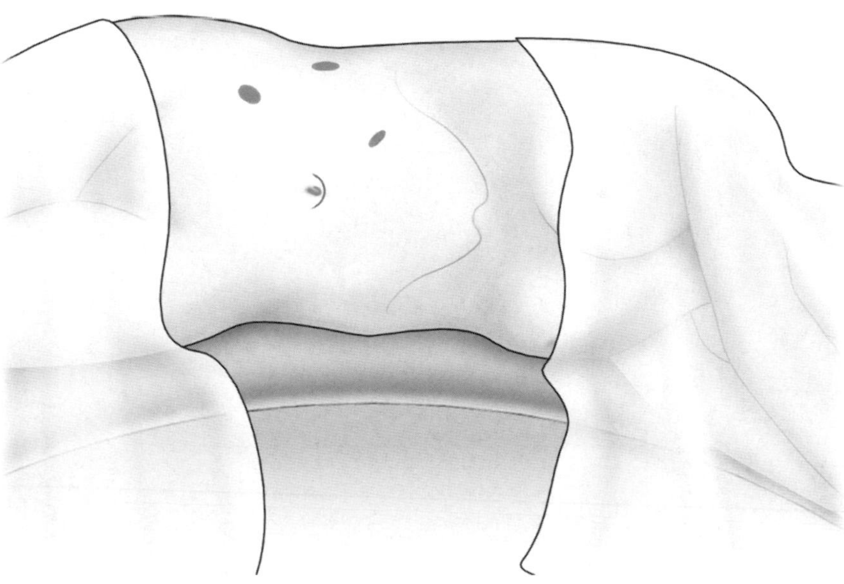

FIGURE 6.2. Port placement for right nephroureterectomy. Depending on the patient's morphology, the trocars can be positioned more laterally

After the ascending colon and duodenum have been completely mobilized medially, the inferior vena cava is exposed and dissected with recognition of the right renal vein. Starting from the right renal vein, the lateral edge of the inferior vena cava is then completely mobilized from the perirenal fatty tissue all the way down to the lower pole of the right kidney (Figure 6.3).

The right gonadal vein should be clipped and transected as part of the en bloc dissection of the specimen and included in the template of the pericaval retroperitoneal lymph node dissection (Figure 6.4; see Chapter 7).

After the inferior vena cava has been completely dissected, the lower pole of the right kidney is then lifted off the psoas muscle and mobilized toward the renal vein. The assistant lifts the kidney, facilitating further dissection of the renal hilum and identification of the right renal artery, which usually is located directly below the renal vein. A right angle dissector is used to circumferentially dissect the renal artery. Once the artery has been adequately dissected, a locking clip is placed to occlude the artery, and further dissection of the renal vein is performed.

The use of a right angle dissector is helpful for artery mobilization. Because the right renal vein is short, an endoscopic gastrointestinal anastomosis stapler may be safer for division than locking clips. Further dissection of the renal artery is easier after the renal vein has been divided. After two additional locking clips have been placed, the artery is divided and the mobilization of the kidney from the psoas muscle is continued cephalad.

In nearly all cases, the adrenal gland can be spared. Therefore, the Gerota's fascia is entered cephalad, and the upper pole identified. The perirenal fatty tissue is transected while sparing the adrenal gland. The next step is the lateral dissection and mobilization of the kidney specimen outside Gerota's fascia. The ureter is identified during mobilization of the lower pole of the kidney, but care should be taken to avoid any ureteral injury that may result in dramatic tumor spillage.

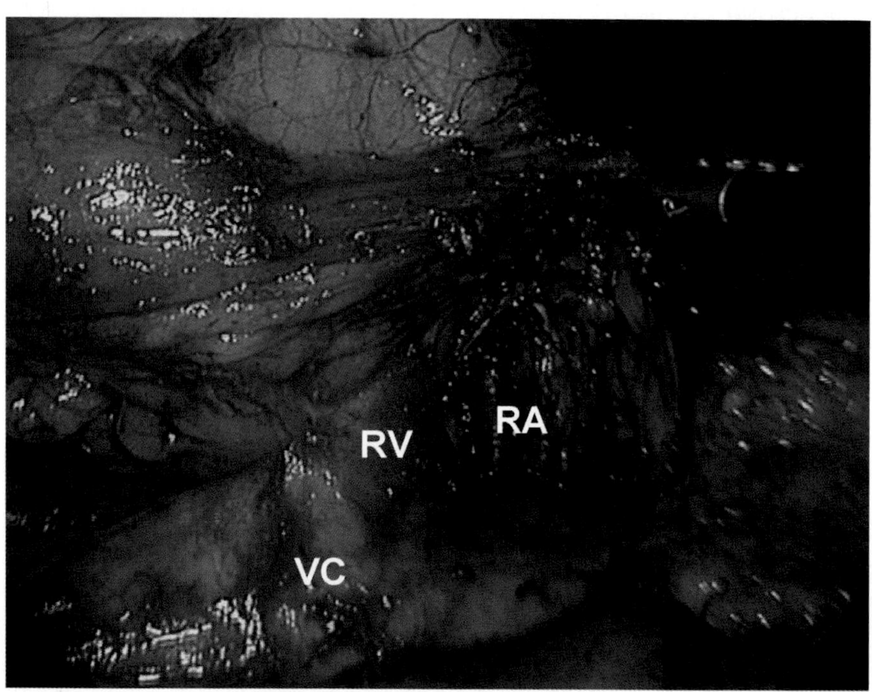

FIGURE 6.3. Dissection of the renal hilum (right side). The dissection of the renal vein (RV) and the renal artery (RA) should be extended toward the vena cava (VC) and the aorta to leave the perihilar structures on the specimen side and initiate the retroperitoneal lymph node dissection

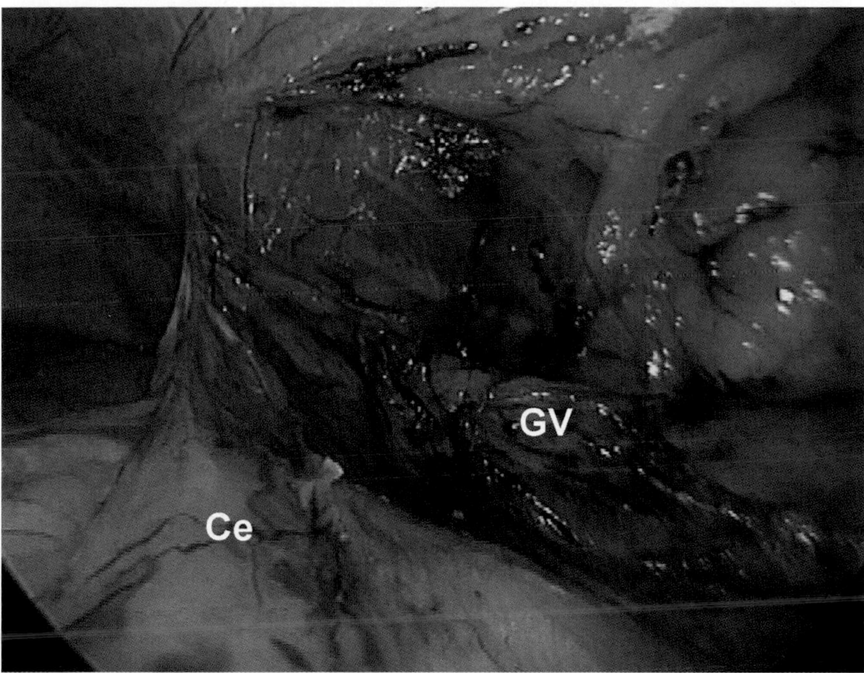

FIGURE 6.4. Mobilization of the ascending colon and the cecum (Ce) to access the retroperitoneum and dissect the gonadal vessel (GV)

After the kidney surrounded by the perirenal fat and Gerota's fascia has been completely mobilized, the proximal ureter is mobilized. The overlying gonadal vessels are clipped and divided, including all the laterocaval structures. The proximal ureter is dissected and mobilized at least until the crossover of the iliac vessels, or even further down into the pelvis if possible.

The entire mobilized specimen is then placed into the pelvis.

A careful inspection for bleeding is performed, and any bleeding controlled with bipolar coagulation. Typically, no drain is placed.

Left Nephroureterectomy

During left nephroureterectomy, it is important to completely mobilize the spleen medially with transection of the splenophrenic ligament. This maneuver helps avoid splenic injuries and helps expose the upper pole of the left kidney. After the descending colon has been completely mobilized, the renal vein can be more easily identified and dissected.

The left renal vein is completely mobilized, including all the branches (gonadal vein, adrenal vein, lumbar vein). The gonadal and lumbar veins are clipped and divided. The left renal vein is raised, and the left renal artery identified posteriorly and dissected. During dissection of the left renal artery, the surgeon is advised to dissect part of the aorta as well for better anatomic identification. After the renal artery has been circumferentially mobilized using a right angle dissector, it is occluded with one locking clip.

The renal vein can then be safely transected between locking clips (two proximal, one distal on the renal vein), and the renal artery divided between clips (two proximal, one distal on the renal artery). The left kidney can then be medially mobilized from the aorta.

The kidney is raised and dissected off the psoas muscle. The adrenal gland can often be spared, by entering the Gerota's fascia at the upper pole and transecting the perirenal fat.

Next, the kidney is laterally dissected outside Gerota's fascia and mobilized. During mobilization of the lower pole of the kidney, the surgeon should

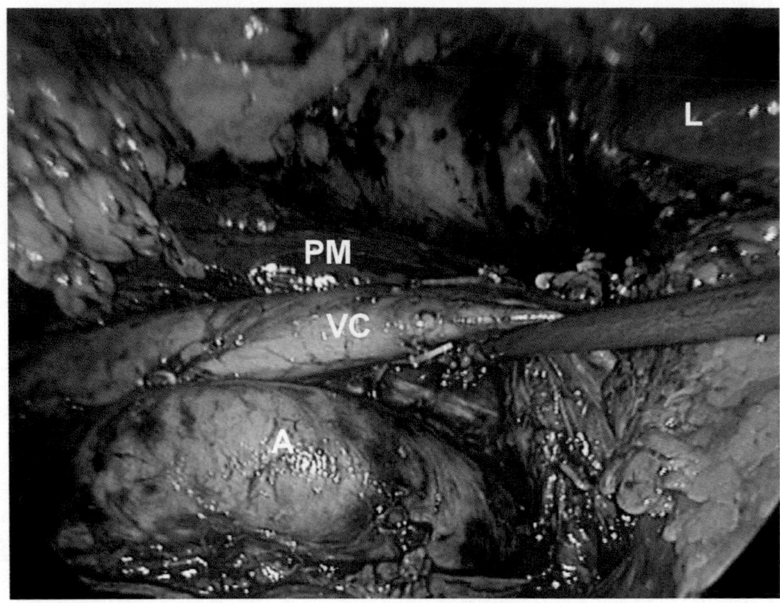

FIGURE 6.5. Dissection of the large vessels and mobilization of the vena cava (VC) to achieve retrocaval and inter-aortocaval retroperitoneal dissection; L = liver, A = aorta, PM = psoas muscle

take care to identify the ureter and avoid injuring it. After the kidney with Gerota's fascia has been completely mobilized, the proximal ureter is mobilized. The overlying gonadal vessels are clipped and divided, including all the lateroaortic structures. The proximal ureter is dissected and mobilized at least until the crossover of the iliac vessels or further down into the pelvis if possible.

At this time, the entire mobilized specimen is placed into the pelvis.

As for the right side, a careful inspection for bleeding is performed. Typically, no drain is placed.

Retroperitoneal Lymphadenectomy

The therapeutic role of lymphadenectomy in transitional cell carcinoma of the upper urinary tract remains unclear. Whether lymphadenectomy is indicated and the extent of lymph node dissection depends on tumor stage and grade. However, in patients with high-grade disease, information about lymph node status is necessary for further adjuvant therapy.

Laparoscopy provides exposure for an extensive retroperitoneal lymphadenectomy and allows removal of the precaval and paracaval (Figure 6.5) or preaortal and para-aortal lymphatic tissue (see Chapter 10).

Management of Distal Ureter

Many different approaches to the distal ureter have been proposed for nephroureterectomy. These techniques often combine features of endoscopic, laparoscopic, or open surgical management. Each technique has distinct advantages and disadvantages, differing not only in technical approach but also in oncologic principles.

The principles of surgical oncology dictate a complete en bloc resection, avoiding any tumor seeding, for all upper urinary tract transitional cell carcinoma. The classical open technique of dissecting the distal ureter and the bladder cuff is recommended for management of distal ureter with bladder cuff resection; the specimen can be extracted later through the iliac incision used to approach the distal ureter.

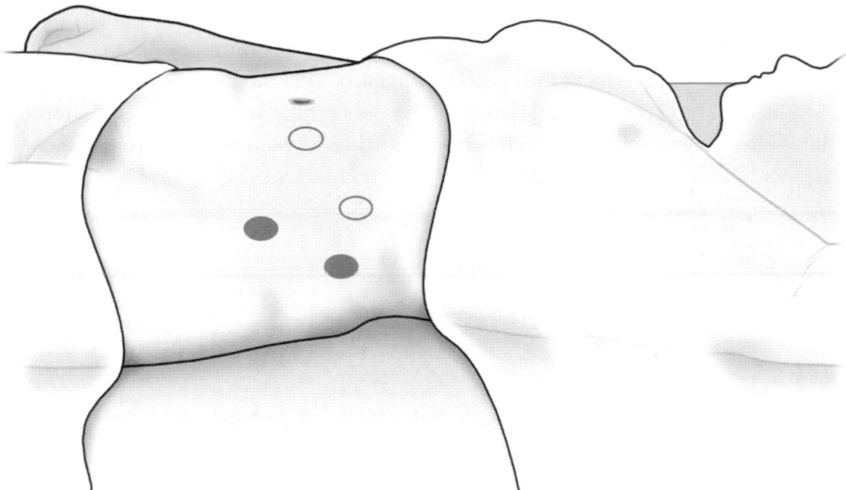

FIGURE 6.6. The iliac incision, starting from the lower port, to dissect the distal portion of the bladder and extract the specimen

For dissection of the distal ureter, the patient is rotated into a supine position as far as the operative table allows. The skin preparation and patient draping performed at the beginning of surgery is adequate for this procedure. A pararectal Gibson incision is performed and continued through the muscle layers (Figure 6.6). After entering the iliac fossa and identifying the iliac vessels, a Bookwalter retractor is placed. The distal ureter is easily identified when crossing the iliac vessels and leads to the kidney specimen. The kidney is extracted and wrapped—a rubber glove may be sufficient—to avoid contamination. The distal ureter is then dissected all the way to the bladder. Therefore, it is necessary to transect the lateral umbilical ligament and eventually mobilize the bladder pedicle. The bladder is op-ened longitudinally between two laterally placed stay sutures, and the ureteral orifice is identified. The ureteral orifice is circumscribed sharply, including a 1-cm cuff of the bladder. The intramural ureter is dissected and mobilized, and finally the entire specimen (kidney with ureter and bladder cuff) is removed.

A two-layer closure of the posterior bladder wall and the bladder incision is performed. The closure sites are tested for leakage by filling the bladder with saline solution (200–300 mL). A Jackson-Pratt drain is placed in the paravesical region and secured before closing the wound.

Postoperative Care

According to the postoperative renal function of the patient, analgesics as well as an oral narcotic can be administered when necessary.

Patients can begin drinking clear fluid on the evening of the day of surgery, with other liquids and foods added according to the patient's progress. A laxative suppository is given on both the first and second days after surgery to help resolve the constipation that commonly develops after transperitoneal nephrectomy.

Discharge by 2 days after surgery is routine, with the bladder catheter connected to a leg bag. The catheter is removed between 5 and 7 days after surgery.

Complications

Potential intraoperative and postoperative complications are identical to those associated with laparoscopic radical nephrectomy. The number, severity, and spectrum of complications depend on the difficulty of the procedure and on the surgeon's level of experience. In addition to the usual complications related to nephrectomy (vascular and bowel injury, see Chapter 4), urinary leakage is a typical and specific postoperative complication of nephroureterectomy.

Because of the wide connection between the pelvis and the peritoneal cavity, a urine ascites could become problematic and cause chemical peritonitis. Continuous drainage of the bladder and pelvis usually results in spontaneous secondary closure. A secondary surgical closure should be considered if urinary leakage is severe and a cystogram reveals a large defect.

7 Retroperitoneal Lymph Node Dissection

Nonseminomatous Germ Cell Tumors

Malignant testicular cancers, both seminomas and nonseminomatous germ cell tumors (NSGCT), can be cured with a very high success rate when correctly managed. For seminomas, retroperitoneal lymph node dissection (RPLND) is rarely indicated. For NSGCTs, which differ substantially from seminomas, the mainstays of successful management are RPLND and chemotherapy, used either alone or in combination. However, RPLND and chemotherapy are both associated with specific morbidities, which increase significantly if the two therapies are combined. Because the therapeutic efficacy of RPLND cannot be further improved significantly, the goal in management of low-stage NSGCT and especially of clinical stage I NSGCT is reduction in morbidity without compromising the cure rate.

Clinical Stage I

About 25%-30% of patients with clinical stage I NSGCT have occult lymph node metastases in the retroperitoneum that cannot be diagnosed preoperatively, even with the most sensitive imaging techniques available. However, in up to 20% of patients whose lymph nodes give suspicious CT results, the pathologic analysis shows stage I disease.

In general, RPLND is considered the only method that can immediately and reliably identify lymph nodes suspected of metastatic involvement without the potential for false-positive results. In replacing open RPLND with laparoscopic RPLND, the aim is to decrease surgical morbidity substantially, while maintaining comparable diagnostic accuracy. The concept presented here, although still debatable, is that RPLND be performed for diagnostic purposes only, implying that treatment for patients with pathologic stage II will be two cycles of adjuvant chemotherapy.

Templates

The specimen to be removed must include all primary retroperitoneal lymph node metastases. Templates described as diagnostic for most clinical stage I patients also contain most metastases in low-stage NSGCTs. The right and left template will contain at least 97% and 95% of all primary metastatic sites.

The templates for the right and left side differ substantially (Figure 7.1). On the right side, the template includes the tissues ventral to the vena cava, the right paracaval and interaortocaval nodes, and the preaortic tissue between the renal left vein and the inferior mesenteric artery. The cranial border is delineated by the renal vessels, and the caudal border by the crossing of the ureter with the iliac artery. The spermatic vessels are removed in their entire length.

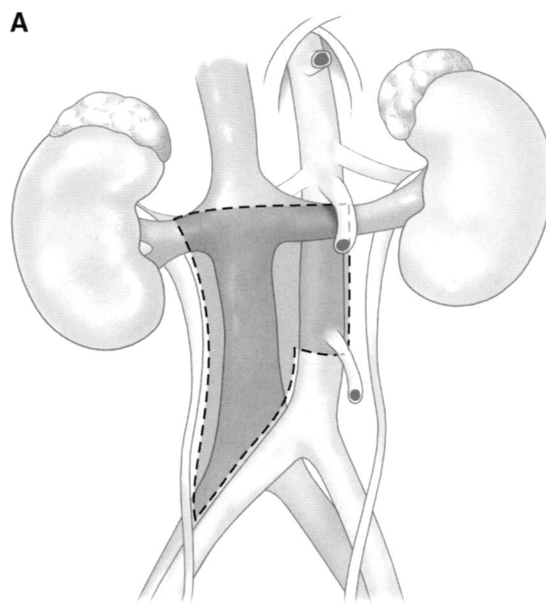

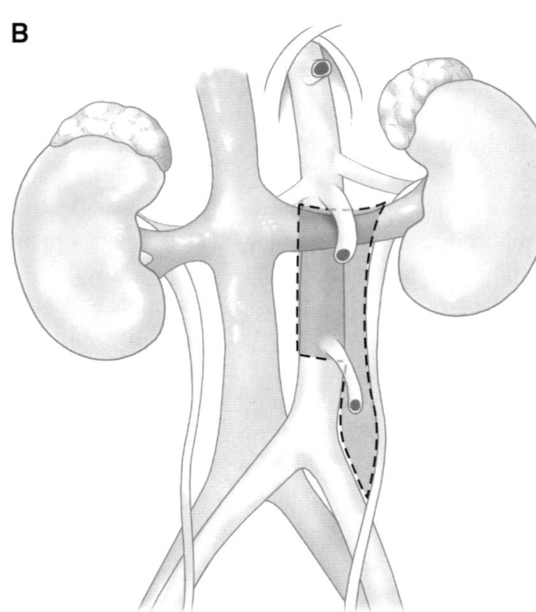

FIGURE 7.1. **(A)** and **(B)** Templates of dissection. A = right side, B = left side

The template for a left sided tumor is somewhat smaller. It does not include the interaortocaval tissue, but includes all tissues lateral to the aorta as well as the tissues ventral to the aorta between the renal vessels and the origin of the inferior mesenteric artery.

In open surgery, within the RPLND template, the lymphatic tissue behind the lumbar vessels must be removed, as well as the lymphatic tissue behind the vena cava and the aorta, to increase the therapeutic value of the surgery. This approach can be reproduced laparoscopically: after the lumbar vessels have been transected, the posterior lymph nodes between the vena cava, aorta, and the spine can be dissected using a "split-and-roll" technique as required in therapeutic RPLND.

The primary lymphatic metastatic sites are thought to invariably be located ventrally, whereas dorsal metastases are thought to result from further tumor spread. So, if RPLND is considered to be a diagnostic procedure only, for clinical stage I tumors, the transection of all lumbar vessels to remove the tissue behind the large vessels might be not required routinely.

Preservation of Antegrade Ejaculation

Loss of antegrade ejaculation is the most common long-term functional complication of bilateral RPLND. This problem can be overcome by performing either a template dissection or nerve-sparing RPLND.

The postganglionic fibers of the right sympathetic nerve travel through the interaortocaval space. The corresponding fibers of the left side are found within the left para-aortic nodes. In a right template dissection (Figure 7.1A), the right postganglionic fibers are resected while all fibers of the left side remain intact. With a left template dissection (Figure 7.1B), all left postganglionic fibers are resected while the right fibers remain intact as long as the interaortocaval space is not approached. Complete unilateral destruction of the sympathetic nerve does not result in loss of antegrade ejaculation as long as the contralateral nerve remains intact. Dissection of the postganglionic fibers is required in bilateral RPLND only, and such a dissection via laparoscopic techniques is feasible.

Contraindications

Contraindications include abnormal values of the tumor markers AFP and beta-HCG. Two other contraindications are uncontrolled bleeding diathesis and pulmonary fibrosis severe enough to prevent pneumoperitoneum.

Obesity or previous surgery does not render laparoscopic surgery impossible. On the contrary, a patient with a high body mass index should experience no more complications than a thin patient, and could benefit from laparoscopic surgery with respect to postoperative pain and morbidity.

Patient Preparation

Bowel preparation, including a clear liquid diet and oral or suppository laxatives, is performed the day before surgery. A low dose of antibiotics is given intraoperatively to all patients for short-term coverage. Typing and cross-matching for two units of blood are routinely performed.

Operative Room Preparation

Instruments

A limited number of specialized instruments are required for this procedure. A mechanical camera holder is recommended to provide stable video images, even in lengthy procedures. For lymphostasis, locking clips are recommended rather than metallic ones, which can fall off easily. However, metallic clips may be required whenever there is a risk that the bulged tip of the locking clips may injure delicate structures. Small surgical sponges held with a 5-mm traumatic grasper are helpful for vessel retraction, and can also be used to apply pressure to stop sudden bleeding (as a substitute for the surgeon's finger).

Patient Positioning

The patient is placed on the operating table with the side elevated 45° upward so that the table can be rotated to place the patient into a supine or lateral decubitus position without repositioning. In addition, the table is slightly flexed at the level of the patient's umbilicus. If necessary, the Trendelenburg or anti-Trendelenburg position is used (Figure 7.2).

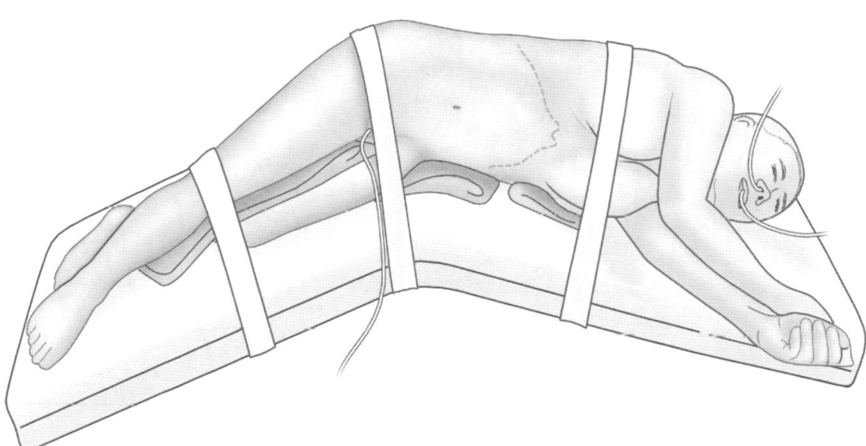

FIGURE 7.2. Patient positioning for dissection of right template

Operative Technique

The procedure is performed transperitoneally. A Veress needle is used for the initial stab incision to create the pneumoperitoneum. Mini-laparotomy and the Hasson cannula are preferred for patients who have had previous abdominal surgery.

Routinely, 10- or 11-mm trocars are used, but one or two of these may be replaced by a 5-mm trocar if desired. The position of trocars is the same for right and left sides. The first trocar for a 30° lens laparoscope is placed at the umbilicus. Two secondary trocars are placed at the lateral edge of the rectus muscle approximately 8 cm above and below the umbilicus. The fourth trocar is positioned in the anterior axillary line to facilitate retraction (Figure 7.3).

Right Side RPLND

Because the templates and the anatomy differ substantially on the right and left sides, the surgical procedures differ accordingly. The templates are described above (Figure 7.1).

Wide access to the retroperitoneum is a prerequisite for RPLND, and wide exposure of the retroperitoneum greatly facilitates removal of the lymph nodes. Therefore, the first step is the most critical. Excellent access is gained by wide dissection of the right colon in the plane of Toldt and of the duodenum.

The peritoneum is incised along the line of Toldt as a first step, from the cecum to the right colonic flexure (Figure 7.4). This incision is then continued cephalad parallel to the transverse colon and lateral to the duodenum along the vena cava all the way to the hepatoduodenal ligament (Figure 7.5). Caudally, the incision is continued along the spermatic vessels down to the internal inguinal ring. Next, the ascending colon, the duodenum, and the head of the pancreas are reflected medially until the anterior surface of the vena cava, the aorta, and the left renal vein at its crossing with the aorta are completely exposed (Figure 7.6).

At this point, the entire template for right-sided tumors is accessible (Figure 7.1). This template includes the interaortocaval lymph nodes, the preaortic tissue between the left renal vein and the

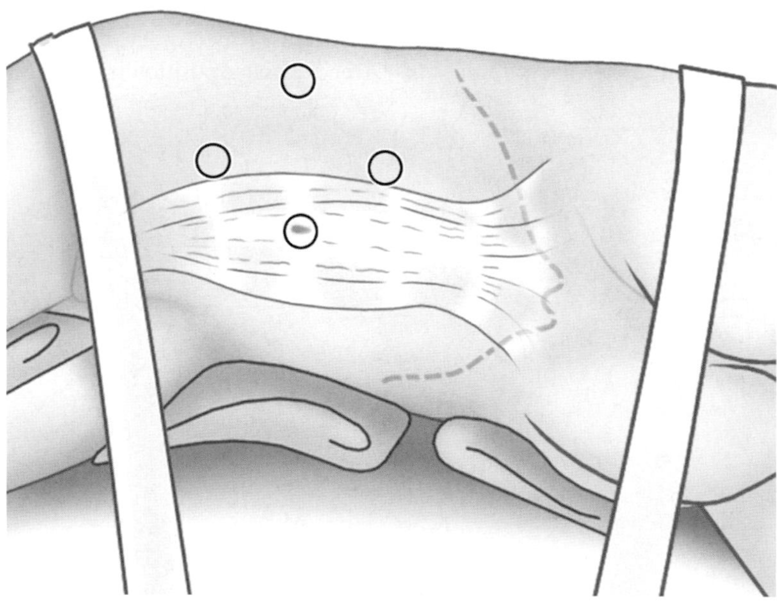

FIGURE 7.3. Right template: a trocar for the endoscope is placed at the umbilicus. Two operative trocars are placed at the lateral edge of the rectus muscle approximately 8 cm above and below the umbilicus. A fourth trocar, for retraction and exposure by the assistant, is positioned at the anterior axillary line

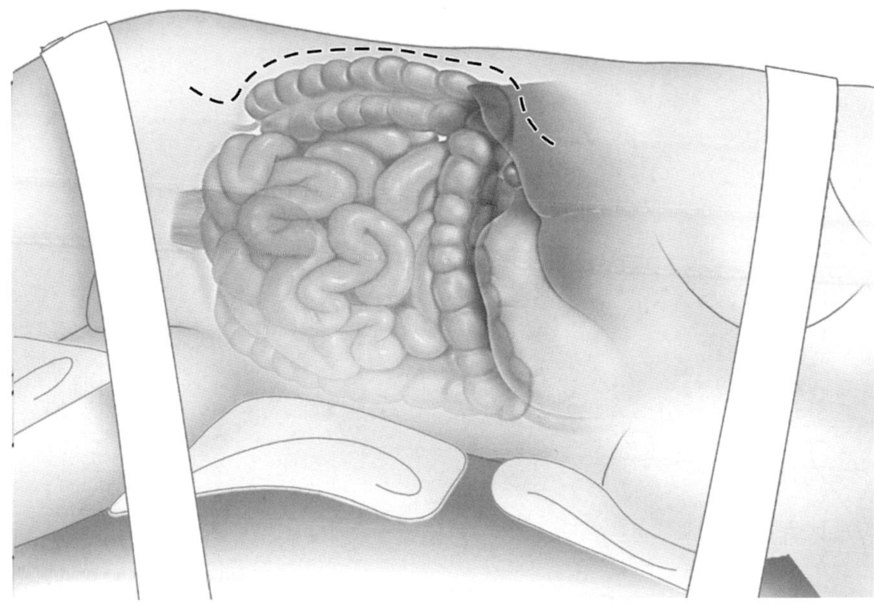

FIGURE 7.4. Right template: peritoneal incision along the line of Toldt to mobilize the entire ascending colon

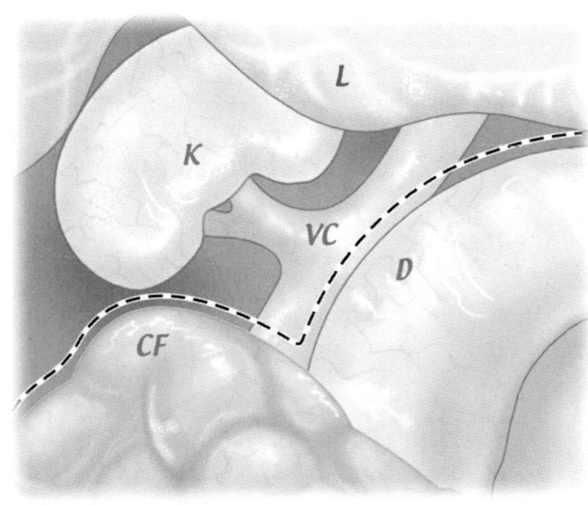

FIGURE 7.5. Right template: anatomy of the right upper retroperitoneum. A peritoneal incision along the vena cava allows the second portion of the duodenum to be mobilized medially (Kocher maneuver).CF = colonic flexure, D = duodenum, K = kidney, L = liver, VC = vena cava

inferior mesenteric artery, and all the tissue ventral and lateral to the vena cava and the right iliac vessels between the renal vessels and the crossing of the ureter with the iliac vessels. The template is bounded laterally by the ureter. Although the dissection does not extend behind the lumbar vessels and the vena cava (and will not be described here), the approach is conceptually and technically similar to that in open surgery.

The spermatic vein is dissected along its entire course starting from the internal inguinal ring (Figure 7.7). Special care must be taken while dissecting its ostium into the vena cava because the vein is liable to rupture at this point. Cranially, the spermatic artery takes a separate course; it is clipped and transected at its crossing with the vena cava; its origin from the aorta is approached later.

The lymphatic tissue overlying the vena cava is then split open from cranial to caudal, and the anterior, medial, and lateral surfaces of the vena cava are dissected free. Both renal veins are freed (Figures 7.8 and 7.9).

The left renal vein is then dissected on its lower border. When the interaortocaval package is dissected in a caudal to a cephalad direction, the left renal vein can be easily injured if it is not clearly visible.

The lymphatic tissue overlying the common iliac artery is incised up to the bifurcation and

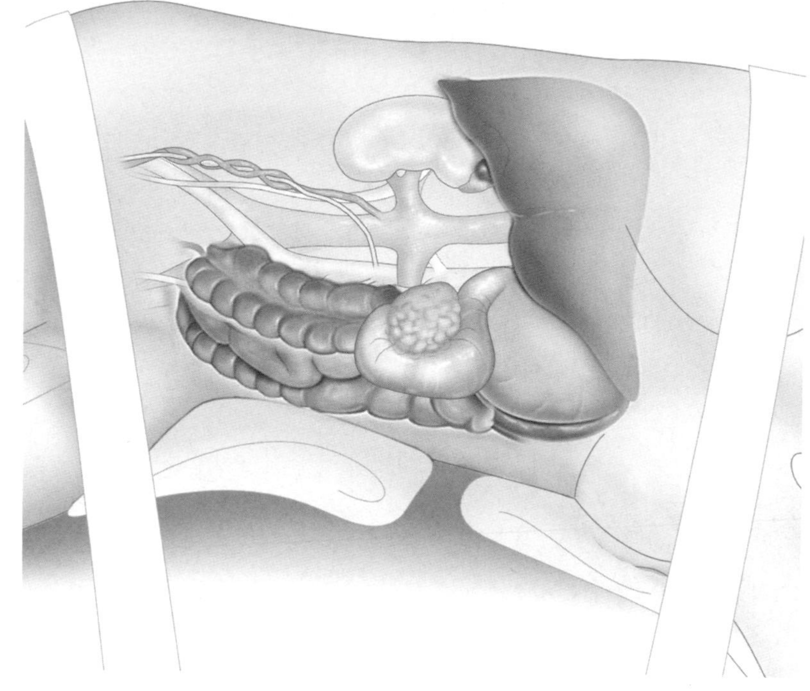

FIGURE 7.6. Right template: exposure of entire right retroperitoneum after deflection of large and small bowel, duodenum, and pancreas

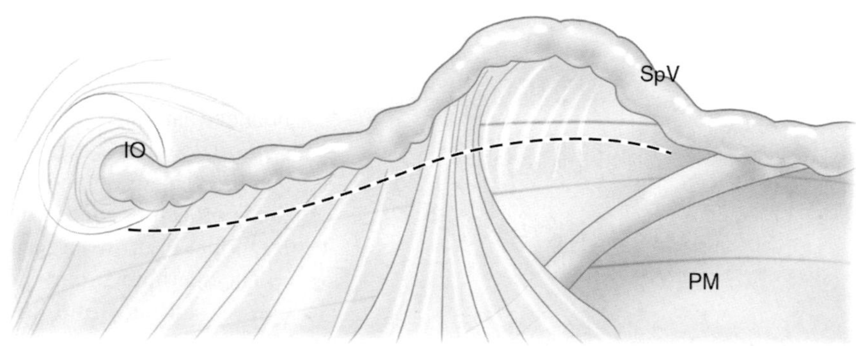

FIGURE 7.7. Right template: excision of right spermatic vessel from its initial ligation at the inguinal orifice. Perivascular tissue should be excised en bloc. IO = inguinal orifice, PM = psoas muscle, SpV = spermatic vessels

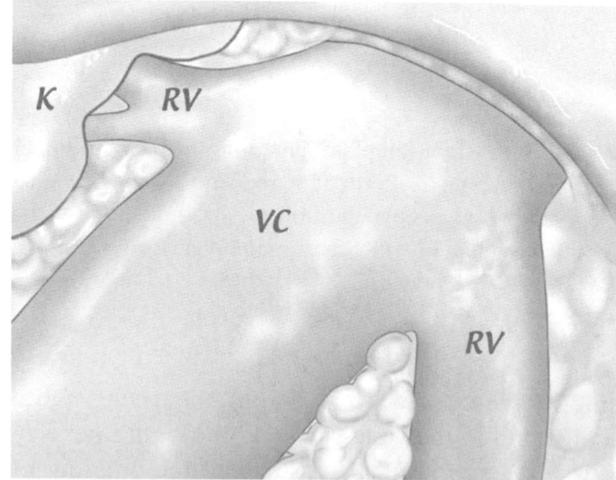

FIGURE 7.8. Right template: vena cava and both renal veins are exposed completely, and the renal veins dissected free. K = kidney, RV = renal vein, VC = vena cava

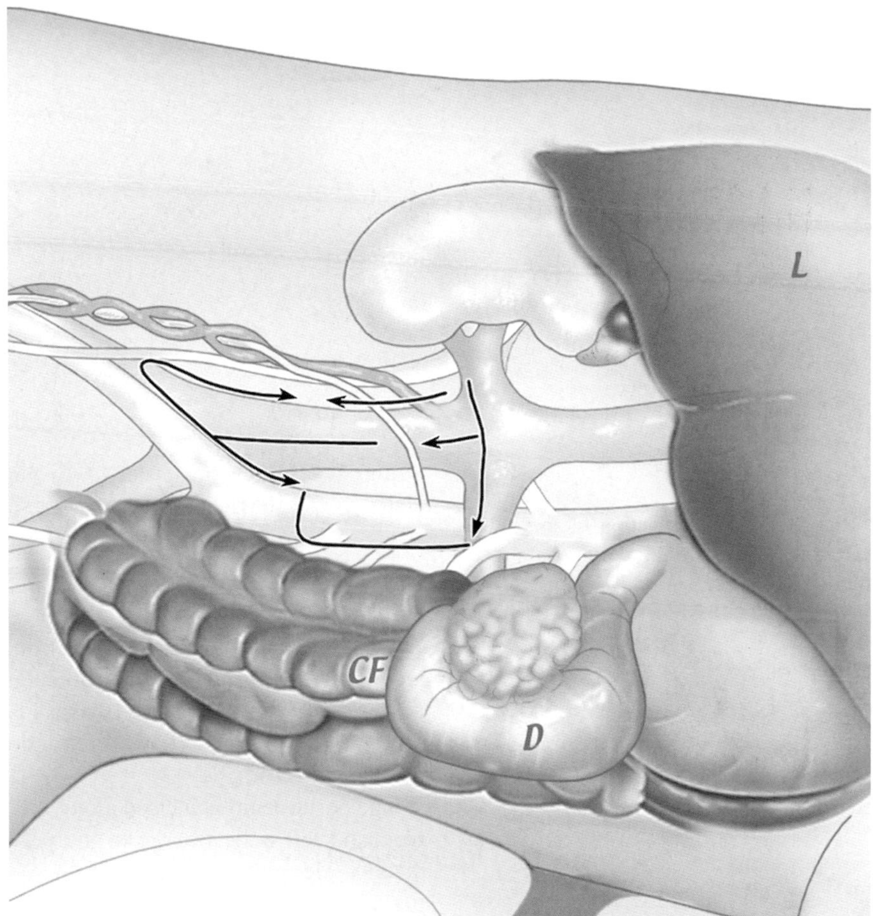

FIGURE 7.9. Right template: intraoperative incision lines in the retroperitoneal space, within the nodal package. CF = colonic flexure, D = duodenum, L = liver

further to the origin of the inferior mesenteric artery. The lymphatic tissue is very dense in this area, and particular care must be taken not to injure the mesenteric artery. Cephalad to the artery, the lymphatic tissue is split along the left border of the aorta so that the ventral surface of the aorta is completely freed. The spermatic artery is then clipped and transected at its origin from the aorta (Figure 7.10). When dissecting the cranial portions of the template, the liver is retracted with a fan retractor.

The right renal artery can be identified at the point that it crosses the interaortocaval space, and the cranial border of the dissection is delineated by the renal artery and vein (Figure 7.11). The dissection is continued down to the lumbar vessels, which are spared, and the interaortocaval package is removed step by step.

The ureter, which defines the lateral border of the dissection, is usually identified during excision of the spermatic vessels (Figure 7.12). It is separated from the nodal package down to its crossing with the iliac artery. This point delineates the distal border of the dissection, where the lymph node package is clipped and transected.

The lymph nodes are then dissected free in a cephalad direction. The lumbar veins are exposed, but they are transected only to facilitate removal of the lymph nodes. Cranially, the ureter enters Gerota's fascia, which can also be differentiated clearly from the lymphatic tissue. In addition to the right renal vein, the right renal artery is exposed

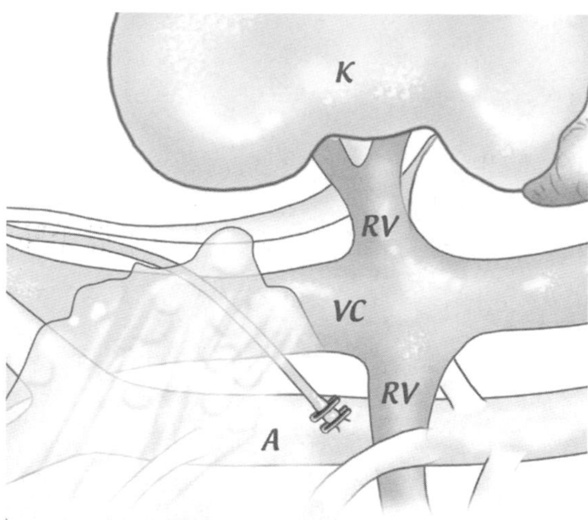

FIGURE 7.10. Right template: dissection of the interaortocaval lymph nodes; the spermatic artery is clipped at its origin from the aorta. A = aorta, K = kidney, RV = renal vein, VC = vena cava

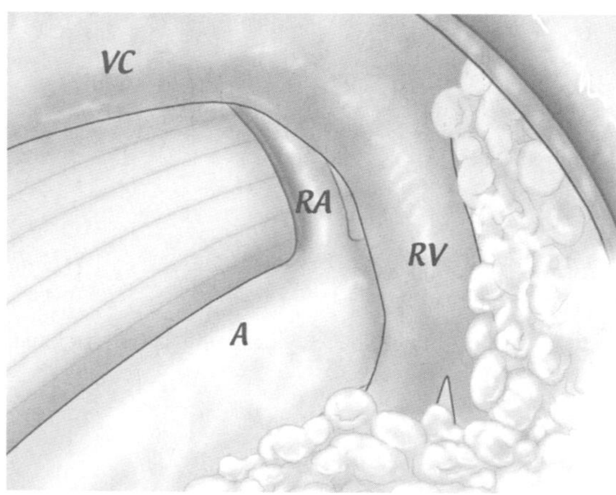

FIGURE 7.11. Right template: upper limit. Interaortocaval space after complete removal of lymph nodes; the right renal artery and the left renal vein delineate the upper border of the right template. A = aorta, RA = renal artery, RV = renal vein, VC = vena cava

lateral to the vena cava, which delineates the cranial border of the dissection in this area. At this point, the nodal package is completely free and can be removed within a specimen retrieval bag. A drain is not placed, because it could facilitate early obliteration of the peritoneal incision, possibly resulting in a lymphocele. Finally, the colon and the duodenum are positioned in their normal anatomic locations and secured with one stitch.

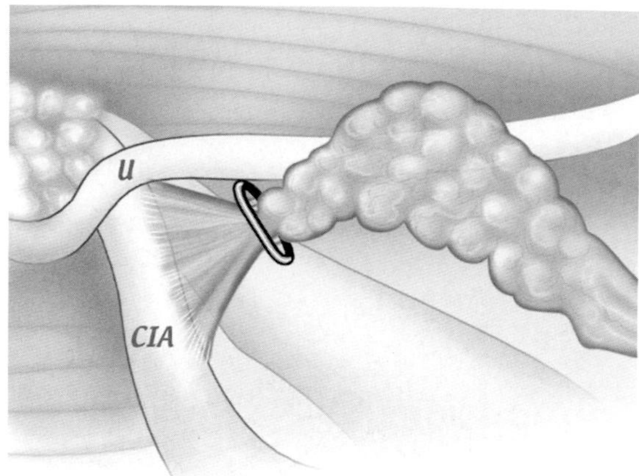

FIGURE 7.12. Right template: lower limit where the ureter crosses the right common iliac artery

Left Side RPLND

The patient is in a right lateral position. The trocars are placed as for right-sided tumors, but in a mirror image array. Usually four 10- or 11-mm trocars will suffice because bowel retraction is rarely necessary.

The peritoneum is incised along the line of Toldt from the left colic flexure to the pelvic brim and distally along the spermatic vein to the internal inguinal ring (Figure 7.13). The splenocolic ligament must also be incised. If the resulting exposure is not ideal, the peritoneal incision is continued cephalad lateral to the spleen up to the diaphragm. The spleen is then completely freed so that it can be rotated 180° medially. This maneuver allows the upper retroperitoneum to become freely accessible. However, this dissection of the spleen is required only in the minority of cases.

The dissection of the descending colon is continued until the anterior surface of the aorta is exposed completely in the plane of Toldt. Normally, the colon falls away from the operative site because of gravity, and a retractor is rarely required.

The spermatic vein is then dissected free along its entire course from the internal inguinal ring to its opening into the renal vein. It is then removed.

The ureter, which defines the lateral border of the template, is identified and separated from the lymphatic tissue. The connective tissue that provides the blood supply of the ureter must be preserved.

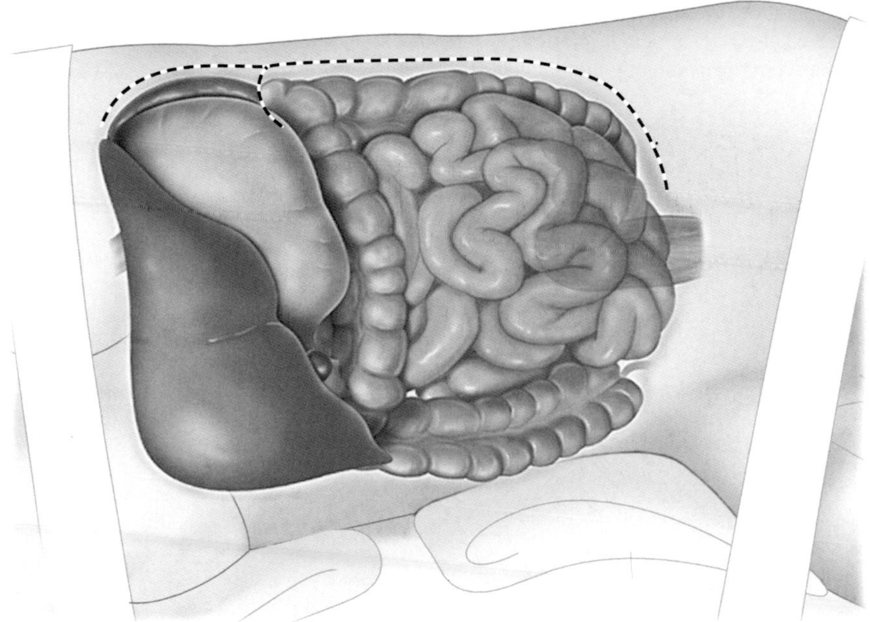

FIGURE 7.13. Left template: peritoneal incision along the line of Toldt and the splenocolic ligament

The left renal vein, including its course ventral to the aorta, can then be freed completely.

The lymphatic tissue overlying the common iliac artery is split open. The dissection is started at the crossing of the artery with the ureter, which delineates the distal border of the template. From there, the dissection is continued cephalad.

The inferior mesenteric artery is circumvented on the left and preserved. Directly above the mesenteric artery, the dissection is continued along the medial border of the aorta up to the level of the renal vein, which has been previously identified (Figure 7.14).

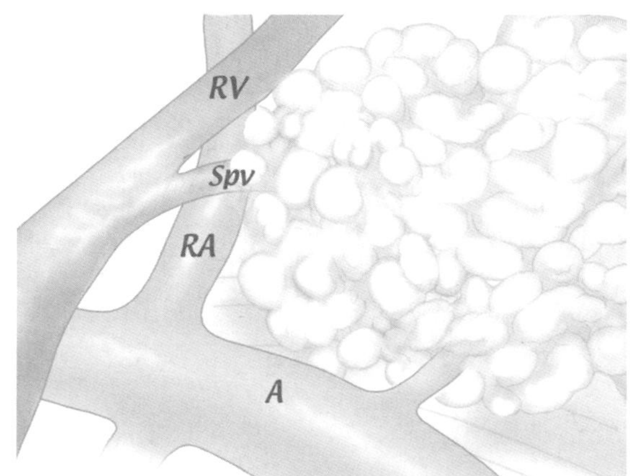

FIGURE 7.14. Left template: upper limit defined by the aorta, left renal artery, and left renal vein at the confluence of the left spermatic vein. A = aorta, RA = renal artery, RV = renal vein, SpV = spermatic vessels

The spermatic artery is secured with clips at its origin from the aorta and transected. The lateral surface of the aorta is dissected down to the origin of the lumbar arteries.

A large lumbar vein is frequently, although not always, present, running between the psoas muscle and the renal vein. This vein is close to the opening of the spermatic vein (Figure 7.15). Sometimes it opens directly into the spermatic vein. This lumbar vein blocks access to the right renal artery. Therefore, it is transected between clips. As a last step, the lumbar vessels are separated from the lymphatic tissue to the point at which they disappear in the layer between the spine and the psoas muscle. The left sympathetic nerve is found directly lateral to this point. The postganglionic fibers, although readily identified in most cases, are not preserved. The nodal package, completely free at this point, is retrieved (Figure 7.16). Finally, the descending colon is placed in its normal anatomic position and secured.

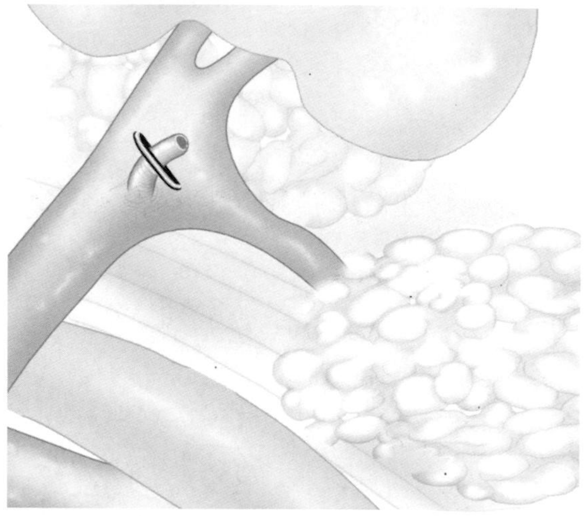

FIGURE 7.15. Left template: the spermatic vein is clipped and transected at the renal vein level; more posteriorly, a lumbar vein opens directly into the left renal vein

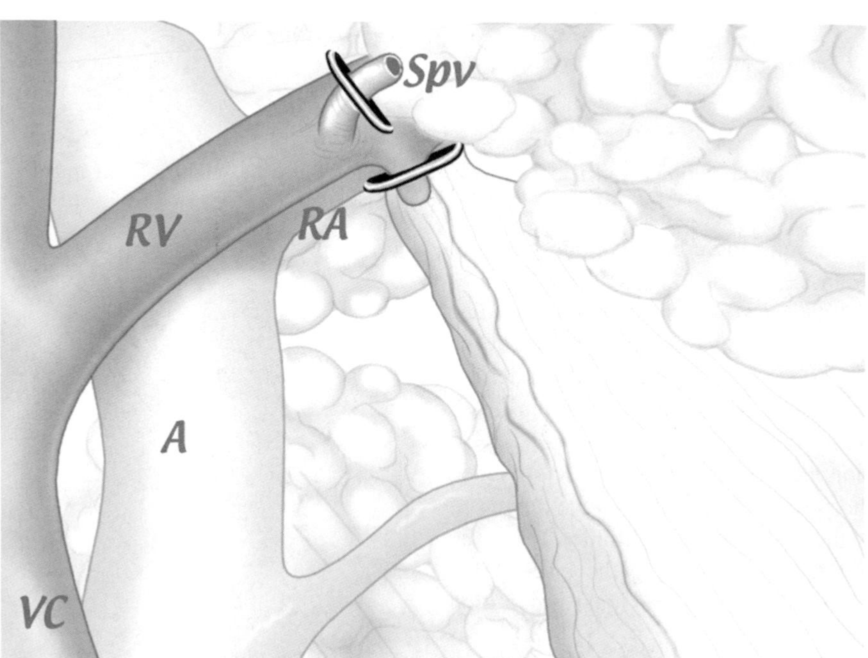

FIGURE 7.16. Left template: the retroperitoneal space after complete removal of all lymph nodes. A = aorta, RA = renal artery, RV = renal vein, SpV = spermatic vein, VC = vena cava

Postchemotherapy RPLND for Stage II

For oncologic more than technical reasons, the size of the primary tumor matters. In larger stage IIc tumors, bilateral tumor spread should be anticipated, and therefore unilateral laparoscopic dissection may not be adequate. For this reason, laparoscopic RPLND is recommended only for stage IIb and in selected stage IIc cases. Whenever unilateral dissection is considered, laparoscopic RPLND is an option. For a complete RPLND, repositioning of the patient from one side to the other is the only way to obtain a total, although consecutive, exposure of the retroperitoneum.

This approach is suitable only for patients whose nodes are not bulky. This surgery can have a high morbidity rate because of many potential complications, mainly vascular, but complications can occur at any step of the procedure.

Surgical Technique

Unilateral RPLND for stage II disease after chemotherapy is performed within the same templates as for stage I disease. Therefore, the technique to gain wide access to the retroperitoneum is essentially the same as that used for clinical stage I disease.

Previous chemotherapy renders identification of the tissue layers more difficult. This problem depends more on the initial tumor size and tumor type than on the number of chemotherapeutic cycles. A mature teratoma is usually well delineated, whereas tumor-free residuals after embryonal carcinoma may be tightly adherent to the surrounding structures. This is particularly true for the vena cava. Small venous branches draining the tumor must be meticulously dissected before they are clipped and transected. A small bipolar dissector as well as a small surgical sponge held by a grasper prove most useful for this purpose.

Postoperative Measures

Chylous ascites is the most frequent complication after postchemotherapeutic laparoscopic RPLND. This complication can be avoided by routinely recommending a low-fat diet with middle-chain triglycerides for 3 weeks after surgery.

Vascular Complications

The most frequent intraoperative complication of RPLND is hemorrhage. Bloodless dissection and adequate hemostasis can best be achieved by bipolar coagulation. Use of the ultrasonic scalpel is not recommended. A small forceps for bipolar coagulation allows for meticulous dissection of delicate structures, whereas broader bipolar forceps provide highly efficient hemostasis.

In open surgery, the surgeon's index finger can be used to instantly stop acute bleeding, while in laparoscopy, a small surgical sponge held with a traumatic grasper can be a good substitute. Once the bleeding has been stopped, the following steps can be performed at a comfortable pace. Additionally, most venous bleedings, including those from small leaks in the vena cava, can be stopped with the help of fibrin glue applied with a dual channel applicator. A strip of oxidized regenerated cellulose or other hemostatic agent can also be used to enhance the tightness of the repair.

As an alternative to tissue sealants, a figure-8 Prolene stitch is recommended. If this is not sufficient, a running suture should be considered, eventually using a locking clip for instance at one end, to gain some time in controlling the bleeding. In most instances, holding the suture under tension after the first stitch can control the bleeding.

As another alternative or in addition to the previous hemostatic techniques, vascular laparoscopic clamps can provide a bloodless field.

If bleeding cannot be controlled by these measures, conversion to open surgery is warranted immediately.

8
Pelvic Lymph Node Dissection

Until recently, pelvic lymph node dissection (PLND) for prostate cancer was performed for diagnostic purposes only. However, for patients with limited prostate tumor bulk and limited nodal involvement, PLND has therapeutic value and may improve the prognosis for long-term survival.

For PLND to be therapeutic, all lymph nodes likely to harbor primary metastases must be removed. The prostate has 3 sets of draining vessels, the most important of which drains into the internal iliac nodes. These nodes are not routinely dissected in limited PLND, which involves dissection of the nodes of the obturator fossa only. Extended PLND markedly increases the detection rate of small solitary lymph node metastases, which means that more than half of the metastases are missed by a PLND limited to the obturator fossa. Because primary lymph node metastases may develop over a much larger region, extended PLND is strongly recommended.

Compared with limited PLND, extended PLND has a longer surgical time and a higher morbidity rate. However, because limited PLND misses at least half of the metastases, the authors believe it is no longer acceptable. If lymph node dissection for prostate cancer is indicated, a more extended node dissection—including the internal iliac vessels, the external iliac vessels, and the obturator vessels—should be performed.

Patient Preparation

A light diet is recommended for about 2 days before surgery and a 12-hour fast before surgery. No bowel or rectal preparation is mandatory, but a Fleet enema or laxative suppository may be recommended, especially for a patient who suffers from constipation.

A single dose of a first-generation cephalosporin should be administrated preoperatively to prevent wound infection, especially at the umbilical site. No antibiotics are indicated postoperatively.

Prevention of deep venous thrombosis is an essential element of perioperative care for patients at high risk of thromboembolic events. Pneumatic compression stockings should be used during and after surgery until the patient resumes ambulation.

Low-molecular-weight heparin is not recommended if PLND is the sole procedure (*see* Chapter 9, Radical Prostatectomy, and Chapter 10, Radical Cystectomy and Urinary Diversion).

No particular preoperative skin preparation is required and shaving is not necessary.

Patient Positioning

The patient is positioned in the dorsal supine position. Thoracic wrap with elastic adhesive tape is used to secure the patient to the table and avoid backward slide with Trendelenburg positioning.

Hard shoulder supports are not used because of the risk of postoperative shoulder pain caused by prolonged pressure on the acromioclavicular joints. Arms are placed alongside the body to avoid injury to the brachial plexus. Hands are protected with mittens to avoid inadvertent injury to the fingers while flexing and unflexing the table.

If the PLND is performed without any other procedures (eg, radical prostatectomy or cystectomy), the legs are left supine; otherwise legs are positioned in flexion-abduction on foam supports after pneumatic compressive stockings have been placed (*see* Chapter 9, Radical Prostatectomy).

Trocar Placement

After a 1-cm radial periumbilical incision, a Veress needle is introduced and insufflation started up to a preset intra-abdominal pressure of 12 mmHg. A 10-mm trocar is then inserted into the umbilicus for passage of the 0° optic.

After ensuring that intraperitoneal injury has not occurred during trocar placement, the patient is placed in the Trendelenburg position, so that the small bowel and the sigmoid colon mobilize cephalad by gravity, facilitating access to the pelvic region.

Four 5-mm trocars are inserted: one into the left iliac fossa, one in the midline halfway between the umbilicus and the pubis, one at the level of the umbilicus in the right pararectal line, and the last one in the right iliac fossa at McBurney's point. The surgical instruments are placed through the 2 ports closest to the optic to have a triangular and therefore ergonomic approach of the instruments. The assistant uses the right lateral and suprapubic ports (*see* Chapter 9, Radical Prostatectomy).

Operative Technique

Template for Extended PLND

The external iliac artery forms the lateral border of dissection. Dissection is continued down to Cooper's ligament. The superior limit of dissection is defined by the bifurcation of the common iliac vessels. The posteromedial limit of dissection is formed by the internal iliac vessels, and the anteromedial limit is represented by the medial umbilical ligament (obliterated umbilical artery).

Again, a complete extended PLND within the template described above is safely accessible only with a transperitoneal approach. Of note, the obturator fossa, corresponding to the limited PLND template, occupies only a small part of the extended PLND template. For bladder cancer, PLND should also include dissection of the common iliac artery up to the bifurcation of the aorta.

Dissection Technique

Monopolar scissors and bipolar forceps are recommended for most of the dissection, because these instruments allow for very delicate tissue handling. Ultrasonic scissors are very efficient and can be helpful when the surgeon is using one hand for retraction and exposure; however such dissection is not as precise as when done with cold scissors and bipolar forceps. Another disadvantage of using ultrasonic scissors is that their active backside can also result in tissue damage from direct contact.

Finally, to decrease the incidence of lymphocele, use of locking clips is recommended to secure lymphostasis of the major lymphatic vessels. Although the transperitoneal approach reduces the risk of postoperative lymphoceles, it cannot be relied on to prevent them entirely.

Peritoneal Incision and Exposure

Wide incision of the peritoneum is recommended (Figure 8.1). The peritoneal incision starts lateral to the medial umbilical ligament and posterior to the vas, and continues superiorly to the level of the internal iliac vessel bifurcation, after the course of the ureter has been identified. If wider exposure is required, as for extended PLND in bladder cancer, the incision follows the course of the common iliac artery.

On the left side, the anatomy is seen differently because the mesentery of the sigmoid colon overlies the common iliac artery and its bifurcation. Therefore, the sigmoid colon must be freed to gain access to the vessels and the ureter. Frequently, adhesions of the large and small bowel have to be released. In this situation, the incision line of the peritoneum must be altered accordingly.

The dissection field is exposed by medial retraction of the medial umbilical ligament with a grasper introduced through the suprapubic port. This retraction opens the virtual space between the bladder and the pelvic sidewall as defined by the internal obturator muscle.

Figure 8.2 depicts the anatomy of the right pelvic sidewall as seen in a frontal view. In thin patients, the ureter can be readily identified before any dissection underneath the peritoneum as it courses over the iliac vessels and medial to the medial umbilical ligament. In all cases, the ureters must be identified because they are the superior landmarks of the PLND template for prostate cancer.

Lymph Node Dissection

The "split-and-roll" technique described for retroperitoneal lymph node dissection (*see* Chapter 7) is used for PLND as well. First, the lymphatic tissue overlying the vessels is incised longitudinally, and the vessels are peeled out of the surrounding tissue. The isolated block of lymphatic tissue can then be released and removed completely.

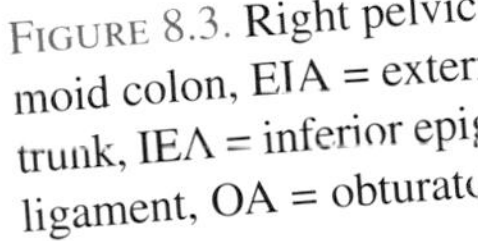

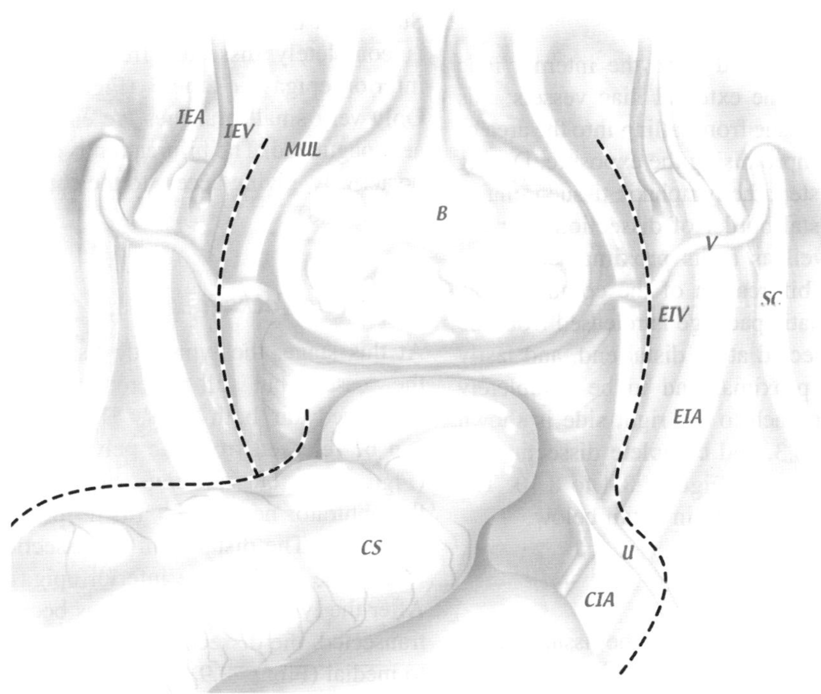

FIGURE 8.1. Laparoscopic overview of the male pelvis. Dashed lines represent the incisions of the peritoneum. B = urinary bladder, CIA = common iliac artery, CS = sigmoid colon, EIA = external iliac artery, EIV = external iliac vein, IEA = inferior epigastric artery, IEV = inferior epigastric vein, MUL = medial umbilical ligament, SC = spermatic cord, U = ureter, V = vas deferens

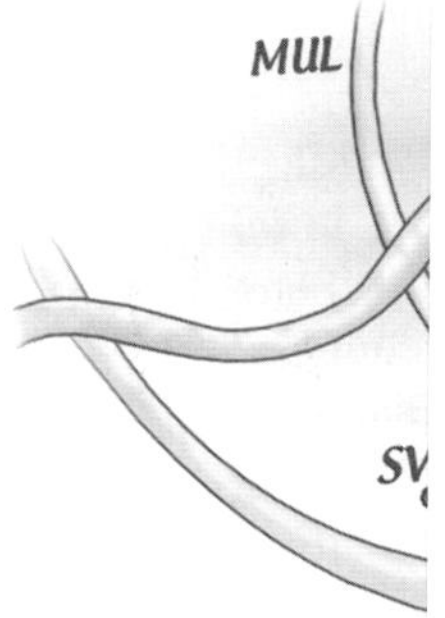

FIGURE 8.2. Fronta
ing the branching c
this pattern are ext
artery, EIA = exter
trunk, MUL = me
tor artery, SGA =
vesical artery, U =

Dissection is
vessels and tov
prevents releas
dissection and
this and the ne
attached at its
pubic bone a
dissection at
artery. The ly
pelvic wall, t
transected at
released. The
in Figures 8
the left side
different ste

Internal Ili

The dissecti
ing the arte
umbilical li
not be freec
sal side by
of the inte

9
Radical Prostatectomy

Patient Considerations

The indications for laparoscopic radical prostatectomy are the same as those for open prostatectomy. However, the laparoscopic approach can be more challenging in certain patients, such as those who are obese or who have a large prostate gland or a narrow, deep pelvis. A history of pelvic fracture, abdominal or pelvic surgery, particularly endoscopic or open prostate surgery, and pelvic radiotherapy can also pose technical difficulties because previous modifications of the structures around the prostate can make identification and dissection of anatomic landmarks less clear. In addition, specific precautions are needed because of the potential presence of adhesions from previous intra-abdominal surgery. For example, the surgeon may consider approaching the dissection of the seminal vesicles anteriorly.

Preoperative Care

A light diet is recommended for 2 days before surgery, and fasting is required for 8 hours before surgery. No bowel preparation is mandatory, but an enema or a laxative suppository may be recommended for patients who suffer from constipation or who are undergoing prostatectomy after radiotherapy.

One dose of a first-generation cephalosporin is administrated preoperatively to prevent wound infection, especially at the umbilical site. Antibiotics are not indicated after surgery or before or after Foley catheter removal unless the patient is at risk of distant infections (heart valves, prostheses, etc.). However, if a cystogram is planned before catheter removal, antibiotic treatment is mandatory.

Prevention of deep venous thrombosis remains an essential element of preoperative care in patients at high risk of thromboembolic events. This includes patients who smoke, who have been in the hospital for a long time, or who have a large prostate gland. Low-molecular-weight heparin, 3500 IU, is administered subcutaneously 2 hours before surgery and every day until discharge.

Operating Room Preparation

Video System and Surgical Instruments

The quality of the video system, especially of the camera and monitor, is essential. A quality camera minimizes the reduction of image quality caused by the anatomic constraints of the pelvis and by minor hemorrhage from small vessels that contribute to the darkening of the operative field. Conventional cathode ray tube (CRT) monitors can still remain superior to liquid crystal display (LCD) panels in terms of color, resolution, brightness, and viewing angle.

Standard surgical instrument packs are sufficient for laparoscopic radical prostatectomy but may be modified depending on surgeon preference and institutional limitations. High-quality bipolar forceps are essential to achieve reliable and accurate hemostasis. Likewise, high-quality needle drivers are important for a quality urethrovesical anastomosis. A suction device with a large inner channel is useful to aspirate clotted blood.

Patient Positioning

The patient is positioned in the dorsal supine position and secured to the table by a thoracic wrap using elastic adhesive tape. This prevents the patient from sliding backward in the Trendelenburg position (Figure 9.1). Hard shoulder supports should not be used because of the risk of postoperative shoulder pain caused by prolonged pressure on

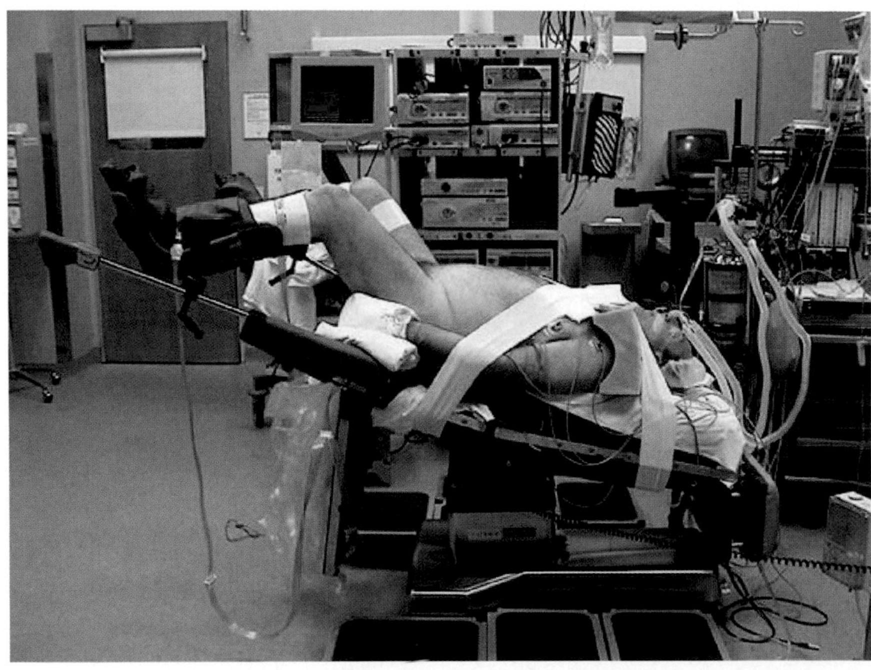

FIGURE 9.1. Patient in Trendelenburg position secured to table by thoracic wrap using elastic adhesive tape; arms placed alongside body, legs positioned in flexion-abduction on foam supports

the acromioclavicular joints. The arms are placed along the side of the body to avoid the risk of injury to the brachial plexus. The hands are protected with mittens to avoid inadvertent injury to the fingers when the table position is changed.

The legs are wrapped in pneumatic compression stockings and then positioned in flexion-abduction on foam supports. Particular attention should be paid to the calves because of the risk of compartmental syndrome. The combination of the increased intramuscular pressure caused by external compression from the calf support (stirrups) and the decreased perfusion pressure caused by the elevated position results in a significant decrease in the difference between the intramuscular pressure and the diastolic blood pressure when the leg is placed in the lithotomy position. This position, along with a long surgical time, can cause acute compartment syndrome. If available, spread bars should be used instead of stirrups.

The open leg position with the buttocks at the lower edge of the operating table (Figure 9.1) is important for two reasons: if the monitor is set on a rolling stand, its location can be adjusted to the surgeon's preference, such as between the patient's legs; and this position allows intraoperative access to the patient's rectum and perineum, if needed.

A camera holder, either mechanical or a voice-activated robotic arm, is hooked to the operating table on the assistant's side, immediately before the patient is secured to the table with elastic bands.

After routine skin preparation, the abdomen is disinfected from the costal margins to the perianal region. Shaving is not necessary. The patient is draped, with the legs covered individually to facilitate access to the perineum. An 18-french Foley catheter is inserted, the balloon filled with 5-10 mL of water, and the bladder drained.

The Surgical Team

A right-handed surgeon stands on the patient's left, with the assistant on the opposite side. Depending on the features of the operating table, the surgeon may need to stand on a surgical stool to be able to operate in a comfortable position, ie, with the shoulders relaxed and the elbows held ergonomically. The scrub nurse stands on the surgeon's left side.

Transperitoneal Approach

Indications and Contraindications

Because the transperitoneal approach has multiple advantages, it is the route of choice. Most important, it allows a thorough pelvic lymph node dissection (PLND). It also offers a larger working space for tissue handling and instrument manipulation. Because the seminal vesicles can be dissected through the pouch of Douglas (posterior approach) before approaching the prostate, their vasculature can be better visualized and controlled. The anterior dissection of the seminal vesicles (ie, after dissection of the bladder neck) is more cumbersome and potentially increases the risk of damaging the nerves that emerge from the inferior hypogastric plexus. Nonetheless, the posterior approach to the seminal vesicles can be technically difficult in obese patients and in those with a large median lobe, and an anterior approach may be warranted in these cases. The transperitoneal approach also allows greater mobilization of the bladder, which decreases the risk of tension in the urethrovesical anastomosis.

Despite these advantages of the transperitoneal approach, the preperitoneal approach avoids the low but serious risk of uroperitoneum (from urinary leakage) or intraperitoneal hemorrhage. In addition, patients who have had multiple prior open abdominal surgeries may benefit from a preperitoneal approach.

Port Placement

After a small (1 cm) radial incision is made around the umbilicus, a Veress needle is introduced and the abdomen insufflated to a preset pressure of 12 mm Hg. A 10-mm trocar is then inserted into the umbilicus for passage of the 0° optic. After the surgeon ensures that trocar insertion has not caused any intraperitoneal injury, the patient is placed in the Trendelenburg position. Gravity pulls the small bowel and sigmoid colon cephalad, which facilitates access to the pelvic region. The height and tilt of the operating table should be adjusted to suit the surgeon's preference.

Routinely, four 5-mm trocars are inserted (larger ones could be used to introduce specific instruments or needles, according to the surgeon's preference): one into the left iliac fossa, one in the midline halfway between the umbilicus and the pubis, one at the level of the umbilicus in the right pararectal line, and one into the right iliac fossa at McBurney's point (Figure 9.2). Operating with the instruments placed through the two ports closest to the optic generally allows the most ergonomic handling of the instruments and is the most comfortable for the surgeon. The assistant uses the right lateral and suprapubic ports.

Alternatively, two working trocars can be inserted symmetrically into each iliac fossa. In this case, the surgeon and assistant operate with their instruments on each side of the optic during the initial dissection of the prostate gland. However, suturing requires the surgeon to use the instruments as described above. Although this approach is far more comfortable for the right shoulder of the surgeon, the instruments are more parallel, making their manipulation less accurate, particularly during the dissection of the left aspect of the gland and deep pelvis.

The Surgery

Pelvic lymph node dissection (PLND) is described in Chapter 8. The technique for laparoscopic radical prostatectomy is described following standardized steps.

Surgical Steps

Step 1: Posterior Approach to the Seminal Vesicles

The posterior approach to the seminal vesicles not only allows their dissection to be more meticulous but also makes the bladder neck more mobile, facilitating its dissection later in the procedure.

Incising the Pouch of Douglas: On occasion, the sigmoid colon needs to be detached from the parietal peritoneal fold to allow its complete mobilization out of the pouch of Douglas and to expose the left iliac vessels in order to perform a PLND. Once mobilized, the sigmoid colon can gently be held by the assistant with the aspiration cannula, retracting the rectosigmoid junction superiorly,

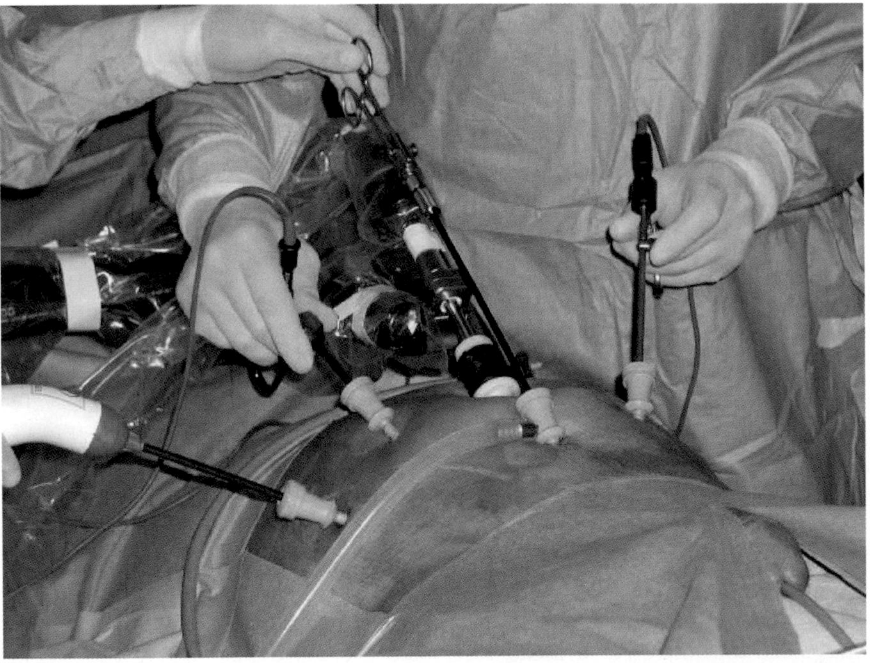

FIGURE 9.2. Port placement—10-mm trocar in place at umbilicus, and four 5-mm trocars inserted as follows: one into left iliac fossa, one in midline halfway between umbilicus and pubis, one at level of umbilicus in right pararectal line, and one into right iliac fossa at McBurney's point. Note that surgeon is operating, while maintaining instruments in triangulation with endoscope

which facilitates access to the seminal vesicles. In thin patients, two peritoneal arches on the anterior aspect of the cul-de-sac of Douglas can be identified. The superior arch lies over the ureters and the trigone. The inferior arch is created by the symphysis of the vas deferens in the midline (Figure 9.3).

The anterior aspect of the cul-de-sac of Douglas must be incised transversely over the inferior peritoneal arch to gain accurate access to the seminal vesicles and the vas deferens. When this arch is not visible, the incision is made about 2 cm above the deepest level of the cul-de-sac. The incision should not be extended more than 4–5 cm laterally to minimize the risk of ureteral injury.

The dissection should then follow the inferior peritoneal flap. After the few subperitoneal vessels have been coagulated, the dissection continues into an avascular plane. This exposes a thin layer of fibroadipose tissue (covering the posterior aspect of the seminal vesicle complex) that should not be confused with Denonvilliers' fascia. Dissecting into this fatty tissue rather than into the avascular plane can lead to damage of either the rectum (dissection too far posterior) or the bladder (dissection too far anterior).

Meticulous hemostasis minimizes the need for use of the suction device, which impairs visibility (by disallowing retraction of the sigmoid colon) and decreases the working space.

Freeing the Seminal Vesicles: Once the layer of fibroadipose tissue covering the seminal vesicle complex has been identified, the outlines of the seminal vesicles and vas deferens (anterior and lateral), covered by the Denonvilliers' fascia, become visible. This sheath is incised transversely to allow clear identification of the vas deferens.

It is usually easier to start the dissection on the vas deferens on either side. The vas deferens is dissected a few centimeters from the ampulla and then coagulated with bipolar forceps, or clamped and transected. The deferential artery runs between the vas deferens and the seminal vesicles, and so will not be visible until the vas deferens is sectioned (Figure 9.4). The deferential artery is large; careful hemostasis is mandatory to prevent serious bleeding both during and after the surgery. Division of the vas and deferential artery allows access just underneath the seminal vesicle. The assistant grasps the prostatic end of the vas deferens and

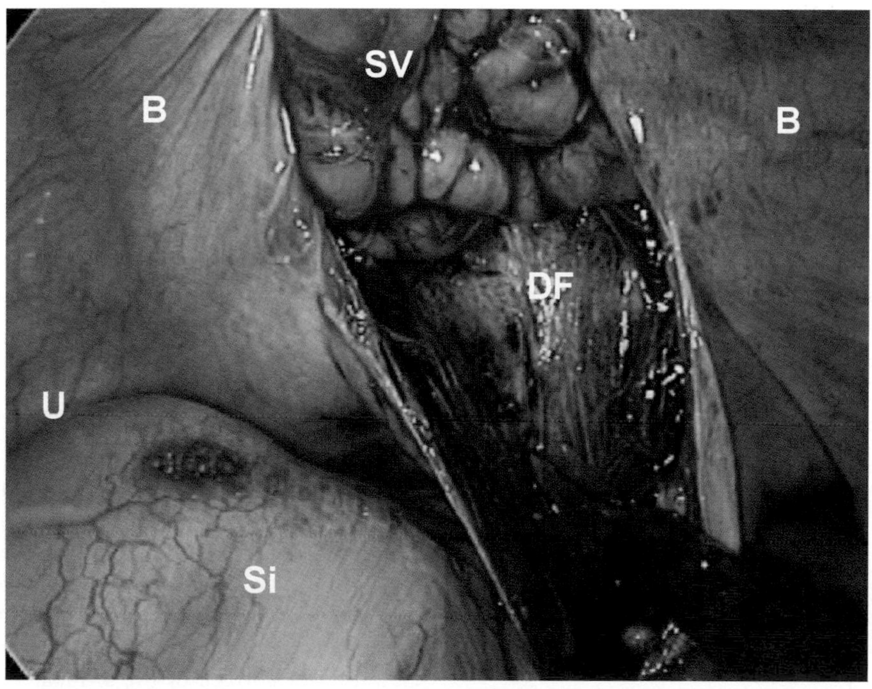

FIGURE 9.3. Posterior approach to seminal vesicles after longitudinal incision of peritoneum on anterior aspect of cul-de-sac of Douglas. Seminal vesicles (SV) become visible after Denonvilliers' fascia (DF) has been incised. B = bladder, Si = sigmoid colon, U = ureter

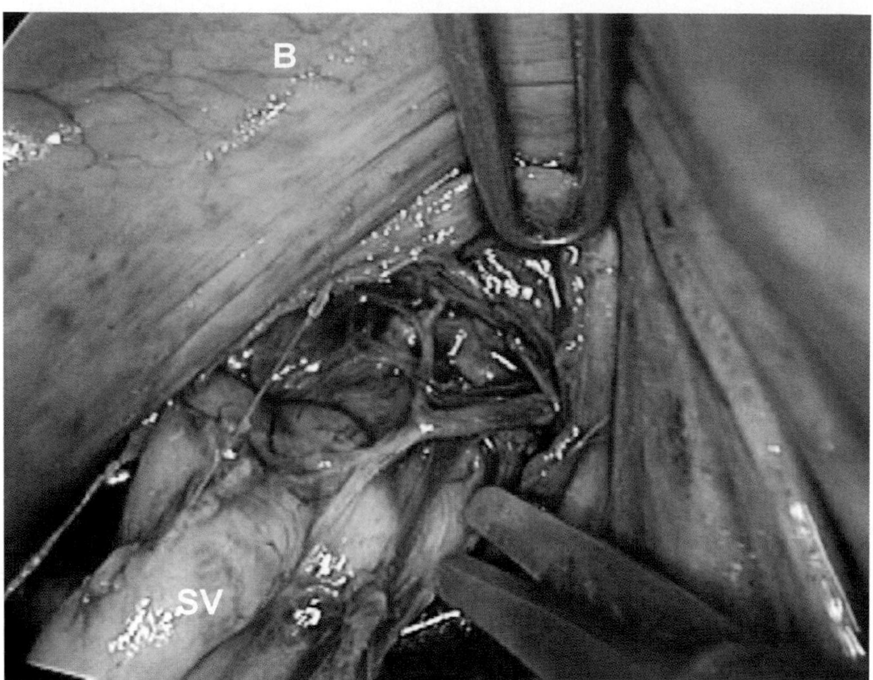

FIGURE 9.4. Dissection of seminal vesicles. Care should be taken in dissecting base of seminal vesicles (SV), where ascending arteries coming from prostatic pedicles could easily bleed. B = bladder

pulls it anteriorly, exposing the posterior aspect of the seminal vesicle. The seminal vesicle should be dissected following a plane along its surface to avoid damage to any surrounding neurologic structures (eg, the inferior hypogastric plexus).

The plane of the posterior aspect of the seminal vesicle is usually avascular or has few vessels, and it can be easily developed. In contrast, the anterior aspect of the seminal vesicle, in contact with the bladder, is usually supplied by one to three arteries.

Dissection of the tip of the seminal vesicle exposes one or two arteries that must be controlled and sectioned to free the seminal vesicle completely. The rest of the seminal vesicle can be dissected toward the prostate without further difficulties.

After the first seminal vesicle has been dissected, the assistant can pull on the previously transected vas deferens to bring the other vas deferens to the midline for its dissection using the same surgical strategy.

Opening Denonvilliers' Fascia: Denonvilliers' fascia must be incised to continue the dissection in the plane of the mesorectum, ie, between the fascia propria of the rectum posteriorly and the posterior aspect of Denonvilliers' fascia anteriorly. This minimizes the possibility of a posterior positive surgical margin.

To incise Denonvilliers' fascia, the assistant retracts both vas deferens upward with a grasper introduced through the suprapubic port to "tent" Denonvilliers' fascia. The surgeon simultaneously pushes the rectum downward with the bipolar forceps introduced through the left port to further stretch the fascia, and cuts it with cold scissors held in the right hand. Denonvilliers' fascia is easily recognized by the presence of longitudinal striations (Figure 2.4). Before incising the fascia, it is often necessary to push it with blunt dissection until the dissection cannot go any further, ie, to the point at which it becomes adherent to the posterior aspect of the prostate. Denonvilliers' fascia is then incised horizontally (1 cm) in the midline, where it reflects between the base of the prostate base and the posterior surface of the seminal vesicles. This shallow incision exposes the prerectal fat.

Lateral extension of the incision on Denonvilliers' fascia should be avoided because it poses the risk of transecting vessels that emerge medially from the prostatic or seminal vesicles pedicles, and any resultant bleeding is difficult to control through this posterior approach. An attempt to develop a plane between the prostate and the rectum posteriorly toward the prostatic apex should be made when the anatomy allows; otherwise, because the rectal wall is also tented, it could be injured during this dissection.

Incision of Denonvilliers' fascia allows for an easier and safer dissection because it detaches the rectum from the prostatic pedicles. This permits identification of three important anatomic landmarks—the rectum, Denonvilliers' fascia, and the posterior aspect of the prostate—later during surgery.

Step 2: Anterior Approach of the Prostate

Entering the Retropubic Space: The coalescence of the medial umbilical ligaments to the anterior parietal peritoneum provides an avascular field for dissection into the retropubic space. The initial point of access is between the medial and lateral ligaments (anterior peritoneal fold on the inferior epigastric vessels) anterior to the vas deferens. Posteriorly, the dissection continues to where the vas deferens crosses the umbilical ligaments (Figure 9.5).

The dissection begins on the right by pulling the right umbilical ligament medially. The anterior parietal peritoneum is then incised in the line where the fat "finishes" and the peritoneum becomes more "transparent." The bladder is incised and pulled backward until the pubic bone or the pubic ramus covered by Cooper's ligament is recognized. Little fulguration should be needed because this is a plane of coalescence. This also keeps the bladder neck facing downward, which keeps it out of the surgical field during dissection of the prostatic pedicles and neurovascular bundles.

Incising either the urachus or the umbilical ligaments is not needed and will only increase both surgical time and the risk of bleeding.

Freeing the bladder wall from its lateral and anterior attachments is essential to create a large working space and to permit a tension-free vesicourethral anastomosis later on. Once the bladder has been freed, it should be completely emptied

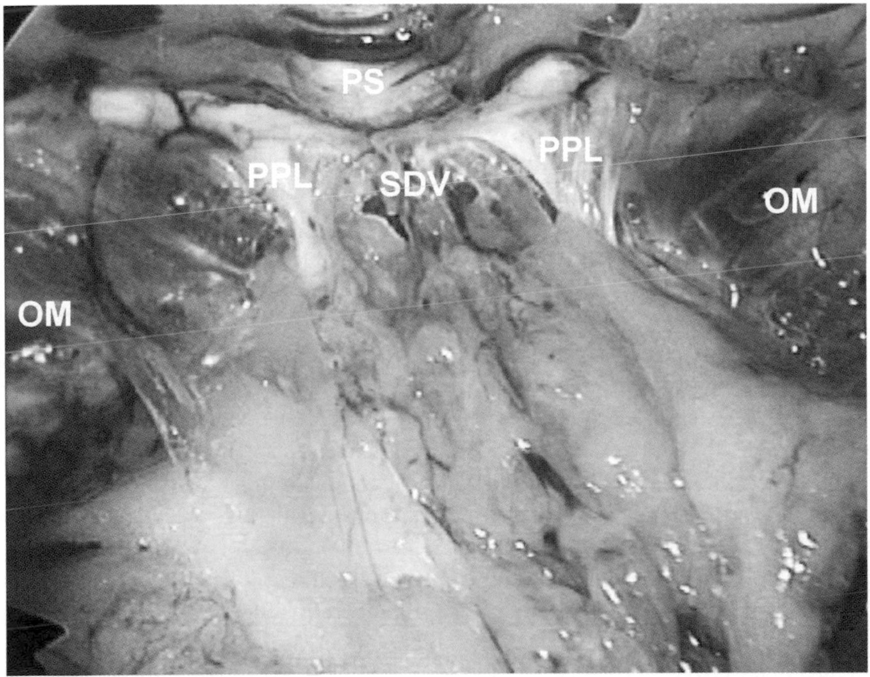

Figure 9.5. View of anterior aspect of prostate after space of Retzius has been developed; superficial dorsal vein (SDV) runs between the two puboprostatic ligaments (PPL) that hold prostate to pubic bone; PS = pubic symphysis, OM = obturator muscle

with a syringe (the Trendelenburg position may prevent it from emptying passively).

Exposing the Endopelvic Fascia: The retropubic fat must be moved laterally to clearly expose the internal obturator muscles, the endopelvic fascia, and the pubovesical ligaments (Figure 2.5). Hemostasis of any tiny vessels within the fat is necessary. This dissection exposes the superficial dorsal vein, which can be easily identified emerging through the pubovesical ligaments. Once this vein is coagulated and transected, the fat covering the endopelvic fascia can be easily moved off to the side.

The entire endopelvic fascia, which is covering the prostate, is incised laterally on its line of reflection, starting at the base of the prostate and extending anteriorly toward the apex. This plane should leave the fascia that is covering the levator ani muscle laterally and the fascia that is covering the sidewall of the prostate. If the periprostatic veins begin to bleed, attempts to fulgurate them are always unsuccessful. It is better either to tamponade the area, or to ignore the bleeding and continue with the dissection. Temporarily increasing the intra-abdominal pressure to 15–20 mm Hg can help tamponade any venous bleeding.

Toward the pubic bone, the endopelvic fascia is reinforced by fibers from the pubovesical ligament, and the levator ani fascia becomes more adherent to the prostatic fascia. Small vessels that penetrate into the prostatic apex or that anastomose to branches of the dorsal vascular complex, as well as apical accessory pudendal arteries, can be identified if the dissection continues toward the apex. While the veins should be fulgurated to allow complete access to the lateral aspect of the apex, the accessory pudendal arteries should be preserved because they may contribute to the blood supply of both the penis and the urethra. Rather than penetrating into the prostate, these accessory pudendal arteries continue their course parallel to the dorsal vascular complex toward the anterior perineum. Small branches of the accessory pudendal arteries that go to the prostatic apex may need to be fulgurated (see Chapter 2).

The pubovesical ligaments are incised at a safe distance from the dorsal vascular complex, as close as possible to the prostatic fascia to maintain the integrity of the suspensory mechanism of the urethral sphincter. This allows the lateral aspect of the dorsal vascular complex, which is covered by an extension of the prostatic fascia, to be visualized. This fascia can be delicately incised to facilitate further dissection and to cleanly expose the lateral aspects of the veins and their inferior limits. (Note also that overdissection of the urethra may contribute to postoperative urinary incontinence.)

If any of the veins forming the dorsal vascular complex begin to bleed, attempts at fulguration are again useless; temporarily increasing the intra-abdominal pressure to 15–20 mm Hg can help.

Step 3: Bladder Neck Dissection

This step can be difficult because the anatomic landmarks are not as well defined as in other steps of the surgery. In addition to being one of the most difficult steps of the laparoscopic radical prostatectomy, dissection of the posterior bladder neck is unquestionably also one of the most crucial because the rest of the dissection depends on how meticulously this step is performed.

The prostatovesical junction must be identified and adequately dissected to minimize the risk of a positive surgical margin at the base of the prostate and to preserve as much bladder neck as possible. The bladder neck should be incised exactly where the fat becomes adherent to the anterior bladder wall (Figure 9.6). To recognize this area, the surgeon must move the anterior prevesical fat superiorly to visualize a faint outline of the prostatovesical plane. (This retraction of the preprostatic fat is possible because the superficial dorsal vein has been previously transected.) The fat tends to be more adherent at the level of the bladder surface (adventitia) than to the endopelvic fascia covering the prostate. The prostatovesical junction should be opened at the level of this adherent fat by transversely incising the prostatic fascia. Several veins run in this layer, requiring careful hemostasis. This maneuver is accomplished by maintaining traction with an instrument on the bladder side, while incising or coagulating fibers and vessels with another instrument (scissors or bipolar forceps). The plane of dissection between the bladder and the prostate is generally easy to develop with alternate sharp and blunt dissection. The mucosa of the anterior bladder neck can be identified by a sudden change in the orientation of the muscular fibers from circular or plexiform to longitudinal. It continues under an “arch” created by the base of the prostate

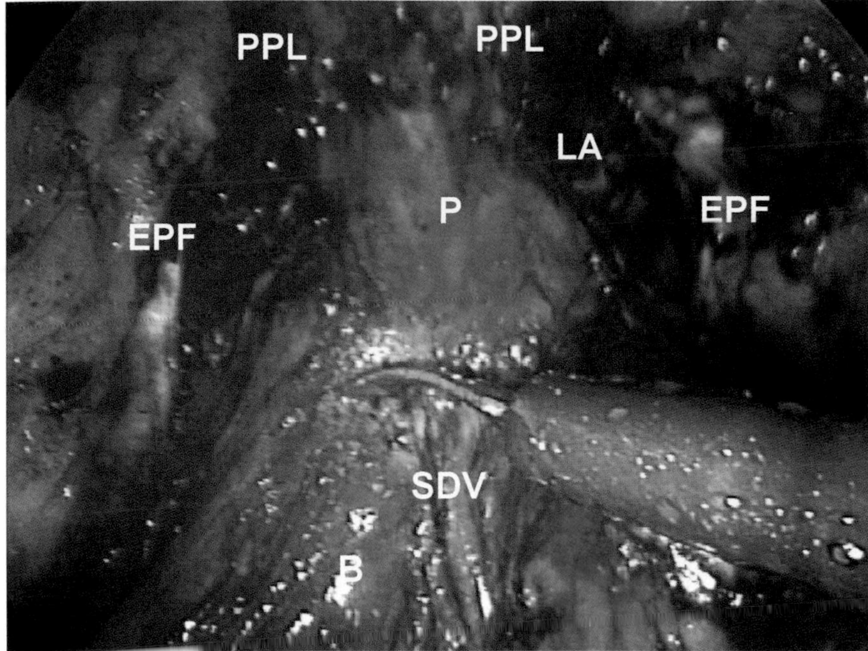

FIGURE 9.6. Bladder neck incision. After superficial dorsal vein (SDV) has been incised, fat covering the prostate (P) can be retracted toward bladder (B), delineating location of incision to approach bladder neck; endopelvic fascia (EPF) is incised on both sides, revealing levator ani muscle (LA); puboprostatic ligaments (PPL) have been preserved

that corresponds to the level where the anterior bladder neck can be safely incised (Figure 9.6). The bladder neck is dissected anteriorly as well as laterally on each side. The bladder is checked again to ensure that it is empty, and the catheter balloon is deflated.

The anterior bladder neck is incised transversely, and the tip of the Foley catheter is pulled upward with a grasper inserted through the suprapubic port. The catheter should be grasped proximal to the orifice to avoid leakage of gas from the pneumoperitoneum. The assistant pulls on this grasper, while also pulling from the catheter to "tent" (i.e., lift up) the prostate, which exposes the posterior wall of the bladder neck (Figure 9.7). The entire thickness of the posterior wall of the bladder neck is then incised. Dissection should proceed slowly because this area is highly vascularized, and discrete coagulation by alternate use of the tip of the scissors and the bipolar forceps is needed.

After the ureteral orifices have been clearly identified, the surgeon grasps the bladder mucosa with a forceps in the left hand and develops the plane with scissors in the right hand. The assistant can improve exposure by gently pulling the bladder neck down with the head of the suction unit. Extending the dissection laterally should provide adequate access to this plane. Conceptually, the goal of the dissection of the posterior bladder neck is to dissect the bladder off the prostate (rather than the prostate off the bladder). The dissection should continue in a straight line following the posterior bladder wall, and not the contour of the prostate. If this plane is confused with the surgical capsule, the plane of dissection will be inadvertently developed between the central and the peripheral zone of the prostate, rather than between the prostate and the bladder. If this occurs, the dissection should be redirected more posteriorly to find the correct plane. Unfortunately, the incorrect plane is very easy to develop and, therefore, appealing. In other words, if the plane is easily developed, it is probably the wrong one.

When the correct plane has been dissected, the longitudinal fascia of the detrusor muscle fibers can be recognized inserting into the base of the prostate (see Chapter 2). The detrusor muscle fibers should not be confused with the rectal wall. Incising the

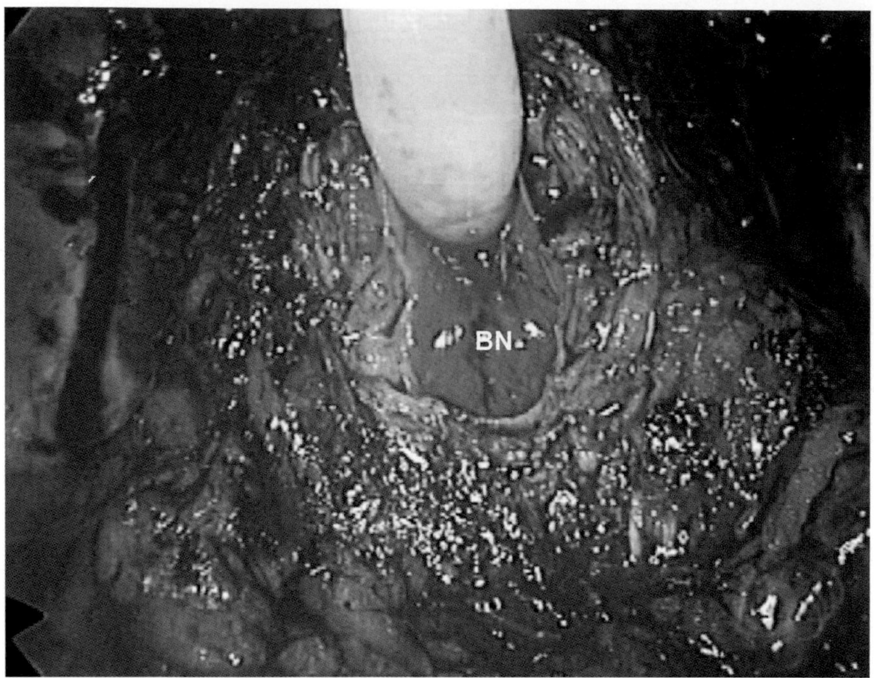

FIGURE 9.7. Bladder neck opening. After bladder neck has been opened, Foley catheter is used to lift up prostate; maintaining tension on catheter exposes posterior bladder neck, facilitating control of trigone and position of ureteral orifices. BN = bladder neck

detrusor muscle fibers at the posterior bladder neck ascertains the correct plane of dissection and provides access to the seminal vesicle complex.

Further intraoperative complications can develop if the correct plane of dissection is missed. If the posterior bladder neck is dissected too close to the base of the prostate, the risk of causing a positive surgical margin at this level is increased. If the base of the prostate is inadvertently incised, arterial bleeding may be impossible to control. If the dissection is performed too close to the bladder neck, either the trigone or the intramural part of the ureters may be damaged.

Incision of the posterior bladder neck does not generally cause much bleeding; however, tiny arteries run in the fibroadipose layer that covers the outer aspect of the posterior bladder neck (distal extension of the adventitia of the bladder), so this step must be done with careful hemostasis (e.g., some form of cautery).

The vas deferens and the seminal vesicles are then simply brought anteriorly, which leaves both prostatic pedicles and the edges of the bladder neck lateral to the seminal vesicles.

Step 4: Control of the Prostatic Pedicles and Dissection of the Neurovascular Bundle

After the vas deferens and seminal vesicles have been brought anteriorly, dissection of the posterior bladder neck is completed to identify the prostatic pedicle laterally. The prostatic pedicle should be dissected and the vessels sectioned after hemostasis with meticulous bipolar coagulation or locking clips. This process is facilitated by anterior traction from either the seminal vesicles or the base of the prostate. Depending on how wide the surgeon is planning to dissect the neurovascular bundle, the prostatic pedicles can be controlled at variable distances from the gland. The amount of periprostatic tissue removed with the specimen depends on the characteristics of the tumor, including its location, Gleason score, clinical stage, and imaging findings, and the patient's serum PSA level. These considerations will lead the surgeon to select one of three methods to dissect the neurovascular bundle (Figure 9.8): the intrafascial technique (between the capsule of the gland and the prostatic fascia), the interfascial technique (between

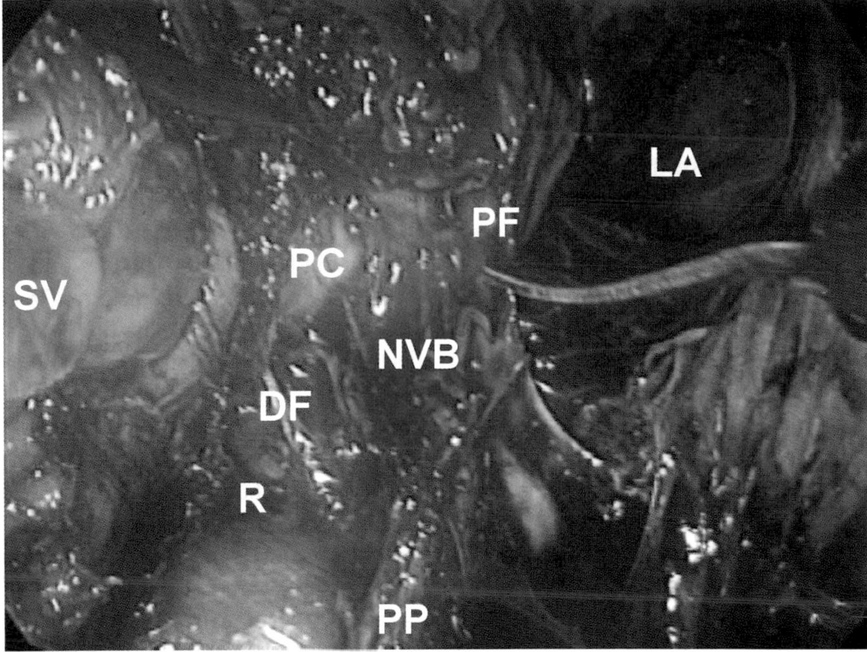

FIGURE 9.8. Initial landmarks of a right neurovascular bundle (NVB) dissection. After prostatic pedicle (PP) has been dissected and incised, prostatic capsule (PC) becomes visible; medial to pedicle, Denonvilliers' fascia (DF) covering medial aspect of NVB is visible and can be incised; laterally, prostatic fascia (PF) is incised on lateral aspect of prostate, when intrafascial dissection of NVB is considered. R = rectum, SV = seminal vesicle (under traction), LA = levator ani muscle

the prostatic fascia and Denonvilliers' fascia), and the extrafascial technique (between Denonvilliers' fascia and the fascia propria of the rectum). In the *intrafascial technique*, the neurovascular bundle dissection follows the plane between the prostatic capsule and the prostatic fascia at the posterolateral angle of the gland. The neurovascular bundle is "completely preserved" and its medial aspect (the side in contact with the prostate) is covered by the prostatic fascia fusing with Denonvilliers' fascia. As the prostate is excised, a layer of Denonvilliers' fascia will remain on its posterior surface, but its posterolateral surfaces (where the neurovascular bundle was located) will be bare of prostatic fascia. In the *interfascial technique*, the neurovascular bundle dissection is performed lateral to the prostatic fascia and includes a slight thickness of the neurovascular bundle. The neurovascular bundle is "partially damaged," and the prostatic fascia fusing with Denonvilliers' fascia remains on the prostate side rather than covering the medial aspect of the neurovascular bundle. In the *extrafascial technique*, the dissection is performed lateral to the neurovascular bundle, which is completely or almost completely resected. Details of each technique are described below.

The Intrafascial Technique: Preserving the Neurovascular Bundle: In the intrafascial technique, the neurovascular bundle is completely preserved by dissecting between the "prostate capsule" and the sheath of fusion between the prostatic fascia and Denonvilliers' fascia posterolaterally. The surgeon should not be able to readily visualize the components of the neurovascular bundle (ie, nerves, vessels, fat) during this dissection.

For a right-handed surgeon, dissecting the right neurovascular bundle first, while standing on the patient's left side, is most comfortable and will allow the prostate to be more mobile during the left-side dissection. The assistant grasps and pulls the vas deferens and the seminal vesicles anteriorly to expose the plane of dissection between the prostate and the posterior bladder neck.

For optimal preservation of the neurovascular bundles, the surgeon must consider three landmarks: Denonvilliers' fascia posteromedially, the

width of the dorsal vascular complex. A "figure-8" stitch is recommended to secure the ligation of the dorsal vascular complex, which can eventually be anchored to the pubovesical ligaments.

Sectioning the Dorsal Vascular Complex: A Béniqué sound is introduced to help identify the urethra by improving the surgeon's ability to both visualize and feel the urethral walls. The dorsal vascular complex is incised tangential to the prostate to avoid a positive surgical margin at the apex, particularly posterior to the urethra. The dorsal vascular plane is divided until an avascular plane between it and the urethra is developed. This plane exposes the anterior and lateral urethral wall, but it should not be developed too widely in an effort to avoid injury to the urethral sphincter.

If the dorsal vascular complex bleeds excessively, using the suction cannula for aspiration will make the bleeding worse. Instead, the pressure in the pneumoperitoneum can be increased to a maximum of 20 mm Hg. The sectioning of the dorsal vascular complex is completed all the way down to the urethra. The assistant holds the previously introduced Béniqué upward to compress the dorsal vascular complex, while the surgeon sutures the avulsion (with 3-0 polyglactin suture on an RB1 needle). See also Complications and Management, p 37.

Completing the Neurovascular Bundle Dissection: The neurovascular bundles diverge from the prostate at its apex, but they must be followed until they enter the pelvic floor, below and lateral to the urethra to avoid any injury. To avoid stretching the urethra and the urethral sphincter, excessive traction should not be applied to the prostate (Figures 9.10 and 9.11).

This neurovascular bundle dissection is performed differently on the right and left sides. In right neurovascular bundle dissection, the grasper is inserted through the left iliac port to grasp the base of the right prostatic pedicle, rolling the gland toward the left and exposing the right distal segment of the right neurovascular bundle. The incision in the prostatic fascia is extended apically, and the neurovascular bundle is bluntly dissected off with scissors inserted through the right paraumbilical port.

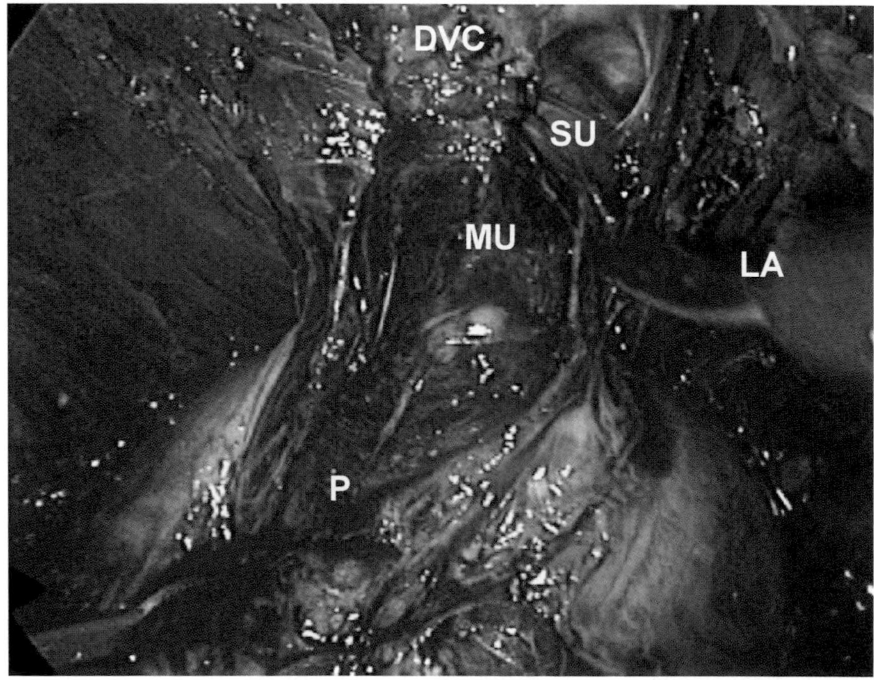

FIGURE 9.10. View of anterior aspect of apex of prostate (P) after deep vascular complex (DVC) has been transected to expose membranous urethra (MU). LA = levator ani muscle, SU = sphincteric urethra

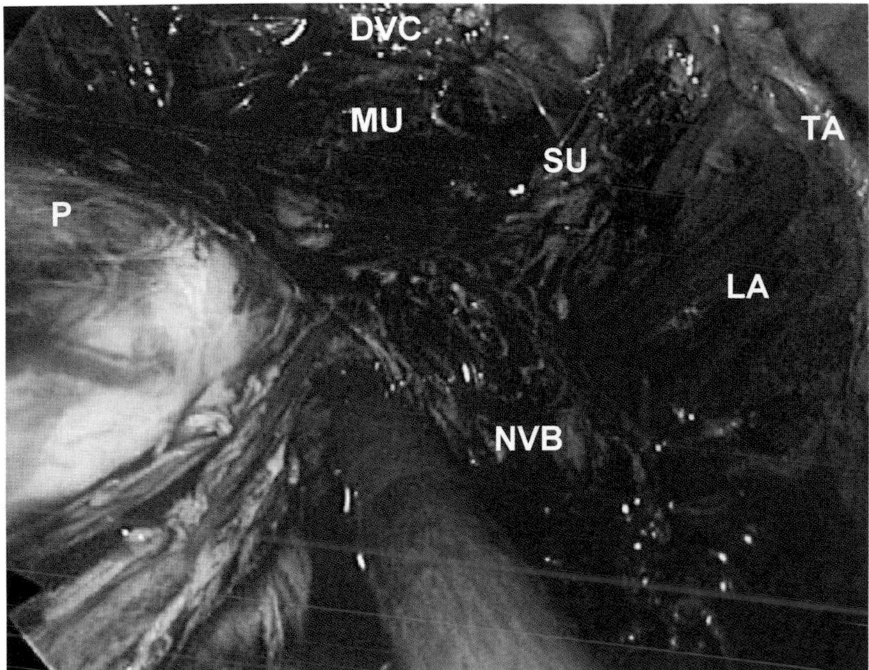

FIGURE 9.11. Laparoscopic view of right lateral apex of prostate (P) after transection of deep vascular complex (DVC) and section of puboprostatic ligaments, demonstrating relationship between membranous urethra (MU), apex of neurovascular bundle (NVB), and sphincteric urethra (SU). LA = levator ani muscle, TA = tendinous arch of levator ani muscle

Visualization of the pulsating cavernous arteries is a good anatomic criterion for anatomic integrity of the neurovascular bundle. Hemorrhage around the bundle is usually minor and, for the sake of neurovascular integrity, should not be fulgurated. However, sometimes, control of one or more apical arteries coming retrograde from the cavernous artery is necessary.

In left neurovascular bundle dissection, the grasper is inserted through the right iliac port to grasp the base of the left prostatic pedicle, allowing the assistant to roll the gland toward the right and expose the left distal segment of the neurovascular bundle.

The surgeon can use forceps through the left iliac port, and scissors through the suprapubic port to obtain the correct angle of dissection. Under certain circumstances, when the dissection space is very limited, the surgeon may need to dissect the neurovascular bundle with scissors in the left hand introduced through the left lateral port.

Transection of Denonvilliers' Fascia: After the neurovascular bundles have been dissected off the apex, the distal attachments of Denonvilliers' fascia are incised. The attachments are separated at the apex and dissected off the posterior aspect of the urethra. Care must be taken not to go all the way across toward the opposite side because this risks injuring the contralateral neurovascular bundle.

Incising the Urethra: Once the prostate has been completely freed, it will hang from the urethra, which should be incised with cold scissors. Sectioning of the urethra at the end decreases the chance of positive surgical margins at the apex by giving a clear view of the junction between the urethra and the prostate. This is particularly important when nerve-sparing is considered.

The specimen is placed into a 10-mm laparoscopic bag, under the control of a 5-mm scope inserted through a lateral port. The umbilical incision can be extended along the midline if needed to accommodate extraction of the specimen and the gland.

The gland is examined macroscopically for induration, nodularity or an area(s) suspicious for positive margin that could require confirmation by a pathologist. If a positive surgical margin is suspected, the entire gland, with the suspicious areas tagged, should be submitted for pathologic evaluation. Evaluation of a possible positive margin should not be done by retaking a sample of tissue from the prostatic bed. If pathologic evaluation confirms a positive surgical margin on the specimen, an additional tissue resection is recommended.

The fascia on the abdominal wall is closed with two running 0 sutures starting at each edge and tightened—but not yet tied—around a 10-mm trocar. The abdomen is re-insufflated and inspected, and any clots are aspirated. The surgical area is irrigated with saline warmed to 37°C. Hemostasis is confirmed. The bed of the seminal vesicles, the prostatic pedicles, and the neurovascular bundle should always be inspected because they are the most frequent sites of postoperative hemorrhage.

Step 6: Urethrovesical Anastomosis

During the anastomosis, the bladder mucosa is never everted. Even when the opening in the bladder neck is large, it is not narrowed before starting the anastomotic suture. In cases of a large bladder neck, an anterior (rather than posterior) tennis racquet is performed at the end of the anastomosis, after the posterior and lateral approximations have been completed.

Throughout the urethrovesical anastomosis, the surgeon works with two needle holders. The anastomosis is made with interrupted stitches of 3-0 polyglactin suture with an #18-mm half-circle needle. The Béniqué sound can help advance the needle into the urethra, taking the full thickness of the urethral wall in the stitch. The needle is progressed into the lumen as the sound is retracted.

Interrupted Sutures: The first four sutures are placed posteriorly from 5 to 7 o'clock, going inside-out on the urethra and outside-in on the bladder neck (Figure 9.12). The 5-o'clock stitch goes inside-out on the urethra (right hand, forehand) and

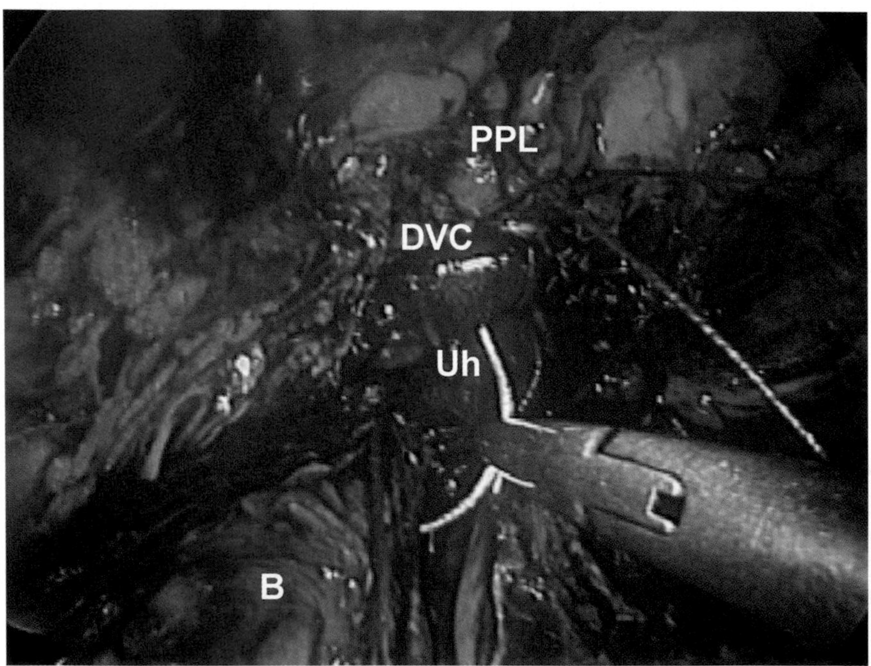

FIGURE 9.12. Anterior stitches of anastomosis with U-stitch placed anteriorly. On right side: outside-in on bladder (B), inside-out on urethra (Uh), inside-out on deep vascular complex (DVC) and puboprostatic ligaments (PPL); on left side: endopelvic fascia, urethra, and bladder, in opposite direction. This U-stitch suspends urethrovesical anastomosis in anatomic position; anterior tennis racket closure with running suture on bladder will complete anastomosis and prevent leakage

outside-in on the bladder (right hand, forehand); the other posterior stitches go inside-out on the urethra (right hand, forehand) and outside-in on the bladder (left hand, forehand). These stitches are therefore tied within the bladder lumen.

Four other sutures are symmetrically placed at 4 and 8 o'clock, then at 2 and 10 o'clock, and tied outside the bladder lumen. For a right-handed surgeon, the right-sided stitches go outside-in on the bladder (right hand, forehand) and inside-out on the urethra (left hand, backhand); the left-sided stitches go outside-in on the bladder (left hand, forehand) and inside-out on the urethra (right hand, backhand).

Three final anterior stitches, at 11, 12, and 1 o'clock, are placed symmetrically to the posterior stitches, with the only difference being that each stitch includes the dorsal vascular complex and the endopelvic fascia. The 11 and 12 o'clock stitches go outside-in on the endopelvic fascia covering the dorsal vascular complex, again outside-in on the urethra and inside-out on the bladder (both right hand, forehand). The 1-o'clock stitch goes outside-in on the bladder (right hand, forehand), inside-out on the urethra, and again inside-out on the endopelvic fascia (both left hand, backhand). After the stitches are tied, a Foley catheter is inserted. The bladder is filled with 180 mL of saline to check that the anastomosis is not leaking and to confirm the correct position of the catheter. Finally, the balloon is inflated with 10 mL of sterile water.

Running Suture: An elegant technique of running suture with a single knot has been described. However, in a running urethrovesical anastomosis, if the urethra is torn at some point, part or all of the anastomosis can become loose and can be particularly difficult to repair, especially at the posterior aspect.

The running suture is prepared by tying together the ends of two 6-inch sutures of 3-0 polyglycolic acid, one dyed and one not dyed for identification purposes. The running stitch begins by placing both needles outside-in through the bladder neck and inside-out on the urethra, one at the 5:30 o'clock position and the other at the 6:30 o'clock position. The sutures are run from these positions toward the 9 and 3 o'clock positions, respectively, using the same maneuvers as described above for the interrupted technique. The posterior lip of the bladder neck is left (1 to 2 cm) apart from the posterior urethra while the first two throws on the urethra and the first three throws on the bladder are completed. Gentle traction is then exerted on each length of suture simultaneously or alternately; the system of loops acts as a winch to bring the bladder in contact with the urethra without excessive traction. A transition suture is completed on either side at the 9 and 3 o'clock positions, by taking an extra inside-out stitch on the bladder. The closure is completed by carrying the suturing up to the 12 o'clock position on both sides, going outside-in on the urethra and inside-out on the bladder. The ends of the running sutures are then tied to one another at the 12 o'clock position on the outside of the bladder.

Difficult Situations

Obese Patients: Several factors make surgery technically more challenging in obese patients. In patients with a body mass index higher than 30, anatomic structure can be more difficult to identify and recognize.

The main issue is proper port placement. The trocars should be inserted higher than usual to compensate for inadequate access and visualization of the apical part of the prostate due to the obstacle of the pubic bone. This different port placement moves the operative field farther away and tends to make the angle of vision and surgical manipulations more tangential to the anatomic structures.

Another issue is additional bleeding that results from transaction of numerous small vessels in the adipose tissue. Progressing slowing and performing careful hemostasis along the way will save time overall.

The patient should always be advised to lose weight before surgery.

Large Median Lobe: The size and the shape of the prostate can also make the surgery more difficult. A large prostate is generally more tedious to mobilize not only because of its weight but also because the angle of dissection to the lateral aspects of the gland is reduced, particularly when the pelvis is deep and narrow. A median lobe poses three additional challenges: gaining correct access to the seminal vesicles (more difficult through an intraperitoneal route), sparing the ureteral orifices, and reconstructing the bladder neck with a secure anastomosis.

In addition, a large median lobe can displace the seminal vesicles posteriorly, radically changing the anatomic appearance of the seminal vesicle complex. This is why starting the bladder dissection right away is recommended in patients with a large median lobe. When the anterior bladder neck is incised, a large median lobe always displaces the Foley catheter off the midline. The bladder opening should be extended laterally to make the "partum" of the median lobe. Placing a transfixing stitch using 3-0 polyglactin suture through both segments of the median lobe and using it to apply gentle traction to enable visualization of the ureteral orifices can facilitate the rest of the surgery.

Difficult Urethrovesical Anastomosis: The urethrovesical anastomosis can be a technical challenge when re approximating the bladder to the urethra is compromised by a short or distal urethral stump. The following steps can be helpful in difficult scenarios: First, perineal pressure can be applied with a sponge stick. Then, if needed, decrease the angle of the Trendelenburg position by 5–10 degrees. If the bladder neck and urethra still cannot be approximated, ensure that the bladder is widely dissected. A final technique is to place traction stitches on both lateral aspects of the urethra, at the 3 and 9 o'clock positions using 3-0 polyglactin on an RB-1 needle. Gentle traction is evenly and simultaneously applied on both stitches while the surgeon starts the urethrovesical anastomosis by placing the posterior sutures. After the first posterior stitches have been tied, the traction stitches can be removed and the anastomosis completed.

If the opening of the bladder neck exceeds the circumference of the urethra, the first rule of thumb is to do a tennis racquet (like in open surgery). However, it should be done on the anterior side of the bladder because doing suturing on the posterior aspect of the bladder neck can be difficult and inaccurate with the anterior bladder neck falling over in the way.

Start the anastomosis (with the preferred technique) without needing to gain any length over the bladder neck. Complete the running suture of the anterior bladder neck opening with 3-0 polyglactin on an RB1 needle. Urine leakage at the anterior urethrovesical anastomosis can be avoided by making the approximation with a U-stitch as follows: bladder (outside/inside) to urethra (inside/outside) to urethra (outside/inside) to bladder (inside/outside). Then the knot is tied, and the tennis racquet is done with a running suture.

The stitch should be tightened with every throw. However, pulling on the suture length should be avoided to avoid simultaneously pulling on the urethra. Holding the suture with one needle holder and squeezing the bladder tissue toward the urethra with the second needle holder will avoid gaps in the suture line.

If the opening is larger than usual, a single traction stitch should be placed at the proximal end of the bladder opening. This can be used not only for traction purposes but also to accurately identify where the opening ends and to tie the running suture.

Urethral Tear: If the urethra tears while the stitch is being tied, no attempt should be made to use the same stitch (that already has a knot in the bladder) or to throw it again through the urethra because the suture can slip when the knot is tied. Cutting that stitch and making a new stitch is always safer.

The urethral stitch can eventually be reinforced by including the endopelvic fascia covering the dorsal vascular complex on the anterior or lateral aspect of the anastomosis. Posteriorly, the urethral stitch can be reinforced by including part of the rectourethralis muscle.

Drain Placement and Closure

The abdominal pressure should be lowered to 5 mm Hg to check for venous bleeding. The peritoneal incisions are left open, and one suction drain is placed through the incision in the pouch of Douglas, between the rectum and the bladder, because this is the most frequent location (left posterolateral) of possible leakage of the anastomosis. A second drain can be placed anterior to the bladder wall through the right lateral port if needed.

The 5-mm trocars are removed, and the parietal orifices checked to ensure that the vasculature, particularly of the epigastric vessels, has not been injured. The incisions are conventionally sutured and dressed.

Postoperative Pain Management

The Three-Step Analgesic Ladder of the World Health Organization to guide analgesic drug therapy is recommended. Patients who have mild to moderate pain are treated with nonopioid analgesic drugs (step 1), such as acetaminophen, aspirin, and other nonsteroidal anti-inflammatory drugs (NSAIDs). Patients taking any NSAID should be monitored for gastropathy, renal or hepatic dysfunction, and bleeding.

If mild to moderate pain persists, the dosage of the nonopioid analgesic is maximized and a step 2 opioid analgesic added. Step 2 opioids used to treat moderate pain include codeine, dihydrocodeine, hydrocodone, oxycodone, and propoxyphene.

For patients who have moderate to severe pain, the dosage of the step 2 opioids can be increased or, if that is not feasible, a step 3 opioid can be prescribed. Step 3 opioids used for moderate to severe pain associated with cancer include morphine, oxycodone, hydromorphone, and fentanyl.

Given its versatility and familiarity, morphine sulfate is generally the opioid of choice in the postanesthesia care unit; however, if it is still required after the immediate recovery period, this should alert the surgeon of a potential underlying problem.

Postoperative Patient Instructions

Patients usually start passing gas 2 days after surgery and have their first bowel movement 3 or 4 days after surgery. Large meals should be avoided until patients begin having bowel movements. Patients are encouraged to drink additional fluids while the Foley catheter is in place, but fluid intake should be decreased to normal (4-6 eight-ounce glasses per day) after the Foley catheter is removed.

The Foley catheter is removed 5 to 7 days after surgery, depending on subjective assessment of healing and the quality of the urethrovesical anastomosis. Kegel exercises should begin within 3 days after catheter removal.

Sexual activity may be resumed 3 weeks after surgery. The patient can resume his normal routine activities 4 weeks after surgery.

Preperitoneal Approach

Indications and Contraindications

The indications for the preperitoneal approach are the same as those for the transperitoneal route. The periperitoneal approach may be beneficial in patients who have had multiple prior transperitoneal surgeries. In contrast, in patients who have had previous preperitoneal repair, particularly when meshes have been placed, development of the correct space could become challenging.

Specific anesthetic considerations are related to the preperitoneal approach because the partial pressure of carbon dioxide is increased to 30–35 mm Hg at the start of the procedure, which requires an increased minute ventilation.

In this book, the term "preperitoneal" is used to refer to an approach in which the peritoneal cavity is not opened. Other authors have used the terms subperitoneal or extraperitoneal, but preperitoneal is the most accurate designation for surgery of the prostate.

Port Placement

Patient Positioning

The patient is prepared in the same way as for the transperitoneal approach. However, the angle of the Trendelenburg position should be set approximately at 20°. In the preperitoneal approach, a greater angle may be needed when there is a breach in the peritoneum to prevent the peritoneal contents from taking up more preperitoneal space and to decrease tension during the suturing of the anastomosis.

Working Space

The procedure starts by making a small (10 mm) incision within the umbilical crease. A similar incision is made on the anterior rectus fascia, and the rectus muscle fibers are vertically separated by blunt dissection with Kelly forceps until the anterior aspect of the umbilicoprevesical fascia is exposed. Finger dissection between the rectus muscle anteriorly and the umbilicoprevesical fascia posteriorly provides access to the retropubic space. This space is further developed with the aid of the optic or, more simply, with the dissecting inflatable balloon.

Creation of Prevesical Space Without Balloon: A 10-mm trocar is inserted through the umbilical incision without preliminary insufflation. The trocar must be directed more tangentially than in the transperitoneal route, placed between the rectus muscle and the arcuate line, or Douglas arcade. The trocar is connected to the insufflation tube, and the carbon dioxide flow is turned on. High-flow pneumodissection occurs spontaneously. The scope is introduced and used to collapse the loose connective tissue to enlarge the prevesical space. The pubic arch is rapidly identified and the tissues are dissected widely on both sides below and lateral to the epigastric vessels to provide sufficient space so that the working trocars can be safely introduced.

Creation of Prevesical Space with Balloon: The balloon trocar is inserted tangential to the cutaneous plane toward the pubis. The optical system is inserted into the balloon trocar to visualize the landmarks of the preperitoneal space during insufflation. This has the advantage of allowing the epigastric vessels to be visualized while the working space is being created. The balloon trocar is then deflated and removed.

An 0 polyglactin suture is then placed in the anterior rectus sheath to secure the optical trocar and to prevent a gas leak. Carbon dioxide is used to insufflate to a pressure of 12 mm Hg.

Placement Sites

The sites of port placement vary depending on the surgeon's preference and on which of the techniques described above have been performed.

If an untreated hernia or unilateral herniorrhaphy is present, dissection can be difficult. In this situation, the first working trocar is placed contralateral to the hernia. The peritoneum is then dissected away from the field with a grasper or adhesions are incised with laparoscopic scissors.

Dissection of the preperitoneal space is completed after the ports have been placed to widen the working space. The location of the peritoneum is checked carefully, and trocars inserted away from it (under direct visualization) because pneumoperitoneum is always a potential source of additional difficulties. Regardless, the thin peritoneum can be damaged, especially in patients who have had previous abdominal surgery (such as an appendectomy). Although this complication can compromise exposure, it does not warrant changing from a preperitoneal to a transperitoneal approach. If peritoneotomy occurs, the following tips can help: the peritoneum should be dissected as high as possible; a small drain catheter can be placed in the left iliac hypochondrium to evacuate excess carbon dioxide in the peritoneum; and the angle of the Trendelenburg position can be decreased.

Initial freeing of the lateral surfaces of the bladder permits better mobility of the bladder to decrease tension during the suturing of the anastomosis. This maneuver can be performed with an atraumatic grasper in the avascular plane anterior to the umbilicoprevesical fascia, dissecting the bladder cephalad and laterally along the external iliac vessels.

The Surgery

The preperitoneal dissection differs in the way the seminal vesicles are approached because they are dissected after the bladder neck has been dissected. Otherwise, the surgery is similar to that described in the transperitoneal approach.

Once the longitudinal fascia of the detrusor has been identified at the posterior bladder neck, it should be incised horizontally in the midline. The ampulla of the vas deferens can be identified in the midline covered by the adventitia of the bladder, which should also be incised. Then, using an atraumatic grasper, the surgeon grasps and elevates one vas deferens. The assistant uses a grasper to retract the bladder for exposure and uses the suction cannula as needed. The vas deferens is dissected a few centimeters from the ampulla and coagulated with bipolar forceps or clipped and then transected. The deferential artery runs between the vas deferens and the seminal vesicles, and so is not visible until the vas is sectioned. Division of the vas deferens and deferential artery allows access to the seminal vesicle on the same side.

The assistant grasps the prostatic end of the vas deferens to expose and facilitate dissection of the seminal vesicles while retracting the bladder posteriorly with the suction cannula to widen the working space. The seminal vesicles are gently dissected to avoid injury to the inferior hypogastric plexus (see Chapter 2). The vessels of the seminal vesicle must be coagulated precisely when they retract after being sectioned. Note that this could be more difficult during this approach than during the transperitoneal one.

Once the seminal vesicles are completely dissected they are pulled up with a grasper by the assistant, and the dissection can continue as in the transperitoneal approach.

The seminal vesicles should be mobilized completely before opening Denonvilliers' fascia and before starting the prostatic pedicle dissection. This avoids injuring the rectal fibers that "tent" when the seminal vesicles are lifted upward by the assistant.

The rest of the procedure is the same an in the transperitoneal approach except that the angle of the Trendelenburg position should be reduced to decrease tension on the urethrovesical anastomosis as it is being stitched.

Robotic-Assisted Prostatectomy

Port Placement

The robot is set up before the patient is brought into the operating room. The system is turned on and performs a self-testing procedure during which it recognizes its spatial position and various components. The camera is black and white-balanced and calibrated. The surgical cart is then draped with sterile plastic sheaths. The following discussion describes only the differences from conventional laparoscopic radical prostatectomy.

Patient preparation is identical to that in the laparoscopic approach. A less steep Trendelenburg position is necessary for the preperitoneal approach than for the transperitoneal route, unless the peritoneum is opened accidentally.

The surgeon operates while seated in front of the master control and looks through binoculars at a three-dimensional image of the operative field. This view is provided by two parallel, three-chip cameras. At the tip of the instruments, a wrist-like articulation enables 7 degrees of freedom for the instruments.

As in traditional laparoscopic prostatectomy, both the transperitoneal and preperitoneal approaches can be used in robotic-assisted prostatectomy.

Usually, this procedure requires five abdominal ports, with a sixth optional port if additional access is necessary or if a second patient-side surgeon or assistant participates in the procedure.

Transperitoneal Approach

The pneumoperitoneum pressure is the same as in the traditional procedure. Three trocars are placed in a triangular pattern. A 12-mm port is positioned at the umbilicus for introduction of the binocular scope. Both 0° and 30° lenses can be used, depending on individual preferences.

The 8-mm port for the left robotic arm (right hand of the surgeon) is placed external to the rectus abdominis muscle. The second 8-mm port for the right robotic arm (left hand of the surgeon) is placed medial to the rectus abdominis muscle.

Two additional ports are placed in the lower left abdominal quadrant for retraction and suction by the assistant, and for the insertion of sutures. One 10-mm port is located between the camera port and the right 8-mm robotic port at the same level as the umbilicus or 1 cm below it. This is done to prevent the camera and the robotic arm on the same side from colliding inside the patient, and also to prevent the assistant's hand and the robotic arm from colliding outside the body. A 5-mm port is then placed laterally and above the left iliac crest.

The robot is positioned, and each arm is docked to its respective port so that any compression or excessive traction of the patient's skin is avoided during the operative movements.

Preperitoneal Approach

The creation of a prevesical working space is similar to that in the traditional laparoscopic approach. In fact, the prevesical working space can be created using a classic laparoscope, which is appreciably lighter than the binocular scope of the robot. The optical trocar is used to dissect the space between the two epigastric vessels and the pubic arch. Forceps are introduced in the trocar that is placed first to create a wider working space. The other ports are placed 1–2 cm lower than in the transperitoneal approach, depending on the size of the patient.

Complications and Management

Intraoperative Complications

Hemorrhage from the Dorsal Vascular Complex

The size and anatomic shape of the dorsal vascular complex varies among patients. A wide dorsal vascular complex in patients with a narrow and deep pelvis is most challenging. Although laparoscopy allows the apex so be seen clearly, and the pneumoperitoneum provides a tamponade effect, bleeding from the dorsal vascular complex can be significant and reduce visibility throughout the surgery. A meticulous apical dissection defining the principal elements around the dorsal vascular complex is essential to prevent unnecessary hemorrhage.

First, all the apical adipose tissue should be dissected off the pubic symphysis superiorly and off the prostate posteriorly and laterally. This brings into view the superficial dorsal vein, which is easily controlled, and provides access to the puboversical ligaments. The latter should be incised close to the prostate side, which widens access to the dorsal vascular complex and allows the periprostatic fascia covering the dorsal vascular complex laterally to be opened. By doing so, the limit between the veins and the urethra is clearly exposed, which facilitates accurate placement of the ligating suture around the entire complex.

When the ligating suture is loose, placed too proximal or cut when the dorsal vascular complex was transected bleeding can be controlled by either increasing the pneumoperitoneum pressure up to 20 mm Hg or by clamping the dorsal vascular complex with a grasper. This allows a tamponade effect while the surgeon prepares a second ligating suture. Undue haste during placement of the second suture may not be successful. Once tied, the suture around the dorsal vascular complex can eventually be anchored to the periosteum of the pubic symphysis to ensure compression and hemostasis.

Bladder Injury

The bladder is most likely to be damaged at three different times during the transperitoneal laparoscopic radical prostatectomy.

First, during the posterior dissection of the seminal vesicles, dissection in fatty tissue should alert the surgeon that the plane of dissection is either too close to the bladder or the rectum.

Second, during the development of the retropubic space, the dissection may be proceeding in the incorrect plane, rather than in the avascular plane. Any excessive bleeding should alert the surgeon that the dissection is too close to the bladder. Filling the bladder with 120-180 mL of saline may help to delineate its walls and to be able to identify any leakage.

Third, during the dissection of the posterior bladder neck, the trigone and the area of the bladder wall under the trigone are at risk. If damage to this area occurs, the surgeon should verify the integrity of the ureters and ureteral orifices and repair the bladder with one layer of polyglactin suture.

Rectal Injury

The rectum can be injured by two mechanisms. The first one is through a rectal tear, which most commonly occurs during the dissection of the posterior surface of the prostatic apex. If not recognized and repaired intraoperatively, the rectal tear will lead to a pelvic abscess and peritonitis. The risk of rectal tear increases when the periprostatic inflammatory reaction is substantial, the patient has had prior prostate surgery or radiation, the patient has a large-volume gland and a narrow pelvis, or a non-nerve sparing procedure is being performed. Inserting a finger into the rectum or a rectal bougie or balloon can help to identify tears as well as to keep surgical manipulations away from the rectal wall during dissection of the posterior aspect of the prostate. While recommendations on early postoperative care (e.g., antibiotics, low-fiber diet, anal dilatation) are similar, management of the rectal injury itself remains a source of debate in regard to interposition of healthy tissue between the rectal repair and the urethrovesical anastomosis versus the need for a diverting colostomy. In the absence of gross fecal soiling, the rectal defect should be repaired with a two-layer primary closure after débridement of any devitalized tissue. While interposition of an omental flap or pararectal fat flap is an added safety measure, it is not routinely necessary. However, in cases of a large, devitalized rectal laceration or gross soiling, a temporary diverting colostomy is advisable.

The second kind of rectal injury is secondary to ischemia of the anterior rectal wall after vigorous dissection or excessive cauterization of vessels on the rectal surface. This devascularization injury cannot be recognized intraoperatively and is frequently manifested by a delayed rectourethral fistula after the Foley catheter is removed. The first therapeutic option is to reinsert the Foley catheter until the fistula heals spontaneously. If this conservative approach is unsuccessful, elective surgical repair of the rectourethral fistula should be considered.

Ureteral Injury

The ureters can be injured either during the dissection of the seminal vesicles by being mistaken for a vas deferens, or by an inadvertent thermal injury. The ureter and the vas deferens can be differentiated several ways: ave multiple differences. First, a ureter that is sectioned will contract and retract, while the vas does not. Second, the vas is in close proximity to the deferential artery, while the ureter is not. Of course, urine will not be seen coming out of a sectioned ureter. During surgery, it is essential to identify the vas deferens and its relationship with the seminal vesicle, from which it is separated by a large deferential artery. If the identification is difficult, the vas deferens is easily approached more laterally as it crosses the iliac vessels and then followed to the level of the seminal vesicle.

If a ureter is mistakenly sectioned and goes unnoticed, uroperitoneum may not develop immediately, especially if the ureter was fulgurated before being sectioned. A persistent urine leakage or uroperitoneum with a watertight anastomosis suggests the diagnosis. Ureteral reimplantation is the treatment of choice.

Another type of ureteral complication is occlusion of the ureteral orifice(s) caused by incorporating the ureteral orifice in the urethrovesical anastomotic sutures. If the ureteral orifice is occluded and anuria and pain develop after surgery, the anastomosis should be redone laparoscopically.

Injury to the Inferior Epigastric Vessels

The inferior epigastric vessels are at risk of injury during port placement. The epigastric artery is most likely to be injured during placement of the right paramedial port. Bleeding, internal or external, around the trocar suggests a vessel injury. Transillumination to locate the epigastric vessels is not reliable; however, in thin patients, the lateral umbilical ligament is an important landmark that can be used to locate the inferior epigastric vessels. Placing the port lateral to the rectus abdominis muscle is safer. Venous injury can be managed successfully by tamponade, whereas arterial injury requires hemostasis by ligation, using a Reverdin or a Carter-Thomason needle. As in all laparoscopic surgery, trocars should be removed while under direct vision and a decreased abdominal pressure.

Postoperative Complications

Urethrovesical Anastomotic Leak

An increased and prolonged urine output from the pelvic drain suggests a urethrovesical anastomotic leak. In most cases, the left posterior aspect of the anastomosis is compromised and can be managed conservatively by leaving the drain in place for additional time. If the leak persists, ureteral injury or eversion of the ureteral orifice unrelated to the anastomosis needs to be considered.

To prevent a severe leak, careful attention during surgery to the posterior aspect of the anastomosis, particularly on the left side, is essential, regardless of suture technique (running or interrupted). The anterior portion of the anastomosis is rarely a source of prolonged postoperative leaks.

Occasionally, a urinary leak is discovered after the catheter is removed. In patients who have had transperitoneal radical prostatectomy, the sudden onset of sharp abdominal pain during or immediately after urination should be considered a urinary leak until proved otherwise. The catheter should be reinserted and the anastomosis reassessed by a retrograde cystogram at a later date to determine if it has healed completely. This "secondary" healing may require an additional 10 days of catheterization, with another cystogram before catheter removal.

A urinalysis should be obtained before any manipulation of the urinary tract if a fistula is suspected to identify and treat any underlying urinary tract infection and to limit the risk of uroperitonitis.

Small-Bowel Injury

The small bowel can be injured during trocar placement or by thermal injury during prostate dissection. An unidentified bowel injury will manifest itself after surgery initially by ileus, mild abdominal pain particularly around the umbilicus, and a normal or decreased white blood cell count. Clinical signs of infection are subtle until the sudden onset of sepsis. Prompt CT imaging with oral contrast can indicate the diagnosis, but a laparoscopic exploratory procedure should be considered if there is any doubt.

Rather than abscess formation, as seen in cases of rectal injury, the clinical picture seen in peritonitis

Indications

Complex ablative and reconstructive laparoscopic surgery begins with careful patient selection with regard to general condition and to the stage of the tumor. In addition, the common exclusion criteria for laparoscopic surgery in general apply. Multiple prior abdominal surgeries, which portend extensive adhesions, usually preclude laparoscopic access; however, prior surgery is only a relative contraindication, and decisions must be made on an individual basis. Obesity must also be evaluated in each individual case. One consideration is the distribution of subcutaneous abdominal fat, which differs among individuals. In patients whose fat is heavily distributed in the lower abdominal and suprapubic regions, traction on trocars to obtain optimal instrument angles may be a limiting factor. As in open surgery, significant obesity may prevent adequate creation of an everted stoma without excessive mesenteric tension. Prior abdominal or pelvic radiation therapy is also a relative contraindication to laparoscopic radical cystectomy and urinary diversion, because massive pelvic fibrosis can be expected. Extensive bladder cancer with infiltration of the bladder pedicles or the pelvic wall precludes a laparoscopic approach; instead, open surgery should be considered for these patients. In any case, with the growing use of neoadjuvant chemotherapy, the typical appearance of infiltrative bladder cancer during surgery can vary.

Preoperative Considerations

Patient Preparation

For bowel preparation, a clear liquid diet is recommended starting 2 days before surgery. Three to four liters of mechanical bowel preparation are administered the day before surgery. Cephalosporin and metronidazole are administered at the induction of anesthesia and for 36 hours after surgery. Heparin (5000 IU) is given subcutaneously and continued after surgery until the patient is ambulatory.

Patient Positioning

The position for cystectomy is the same as that for other laparoscopic pelvic surgery (see Chapter 8, Pelvic Lymph Node Dissection, and Chapter 9, Radical Prostatectomy). Compressive devices are applied to the lower extremities before anesthesia is induced. After the endotracheal tube has been inserted, the patient's stomach is decompressed with a nasogastric tube.

The patient is carefully positioned in the supine position. If a Mainz pouch II diversion is planned, the legs of both male and female patients are placed in a modified lithotomy position to allow access to the perineum. All bony prominences must be padded. Finally, the patient is secured onto the table with straps over the chest and over the legs for additional safety during Trendelenburg positioning and rotation of the table.

The Foley catheter is placed sterilely after the patient has been draped so that it can be accessed during surgery.

Operating Room Preparation

As during laparoscopic radical prostatectomy, the right-handed surgeon and the assisting nurse stand to the patient's left, while the first assistant and the camera holder (an assistant or a mechanical device) are positioned on the patient's right. Monitors are positioned at the level of the patient's feet (between the legs), as are other needed devices (e.e.g, insufflator, light source, suction, etc), which are all on a transportable tower.

The instruments used for laparoscopic radical cystectomy are similar to those used during laparoscopic radical prostatectomy or other pelvic procedures. The particular instruments used depend on the surgeon's preference. Using a bipolar grasper in the left hand and monopolar scissors in the right hand is often recommended for the entire dissection, as it is for all pelvic surgery.

Operative Technique of Radical Cystectomy

Radical Cystectomy in Men

Transperitoneal Access and Port Placement

After an infraumbilical incision has been made, a Veress needle is introduced to obtain a pneumoperitoneum up to 15 mm Hg. A primary 10-mm

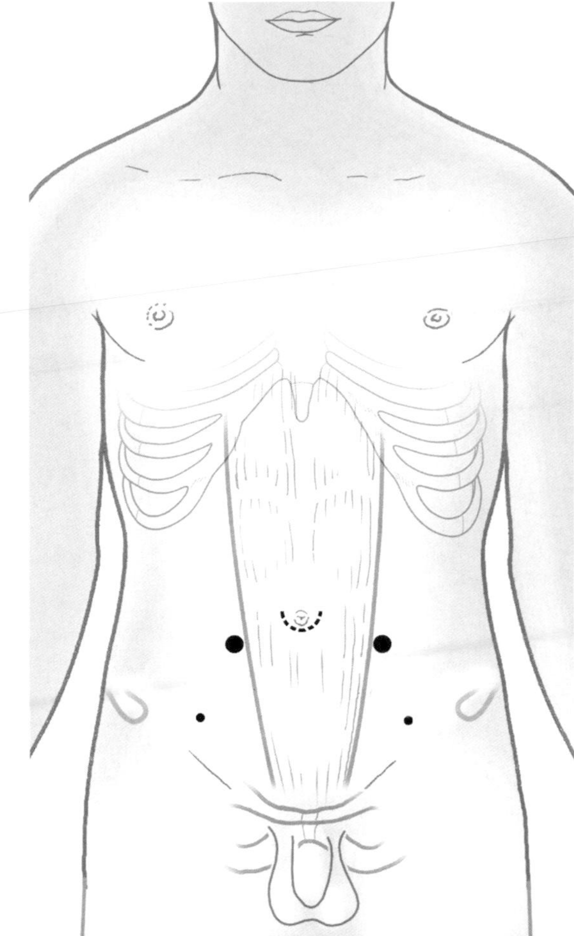

FIGURE 10.1. Number and placement of trocars. A 10-mm laparoscopic trocar for the endoscope is placed at the level of the umbilicus. Four trocars are placed in a fan-shaped array: two 10-mm trocars on the lateral pararectal lines about 10 cm above the pubic symphysis; two 5-mm trocars at 2-3 cm medial to the anterior-superior iliac spine on each side

laparoscopic trocar is placed at the level of the umbilicus. The abdominal cavity is inspected, and the other four trocars are placed in a fan-shaped array. Two 10-mm trocars are placed (under laparoscopic control) on the lateral pararectal lines about 10 cm above the pubic symphysis. Two 5-mm trocars are positioned bilaterally 2-3 cm medial to the anterosuperior iliac spine (Figure 10.1).

After the trocars have been placed, the patient is placed in a steep Trendelenburg position.

Posterior Dissection and Bladder Pedicle Exposure

This step is similar to that in radical prostatectomy (see Chapter 9). The peritoneum is incised at the level of the pouch of Douglas (Figure 10.2). The tips of the seminal vesicles are dissected to expose Denonvilliers' fascia. The fascia is incised in the midline to expose the perirectal fat. The fibers of the rectum are bluntly pushed posteriorly, away from the prostate. This dissection is continued as far as is safely possible toward the apex of the prostate (Figure 10.3). Complete mobilization of the rectum is essential to better define the prostatic and vesical pedicles and to prevent rectal injuries.

Incision of the peritoneum is continued along the course of the external iliac artery and extended distally to the abdominal wall lateral to the umbilical ligaments, and proximally to the common iliac artery (Figure 10.4). At the level of the pubic bone, the bladder and perivesical fat are dissected off the pelvic wall with exposure of the endopelvic fascia. The fascia is incised bilaterally, and the fibers of the levator muscle carefully dissected. This maneuver

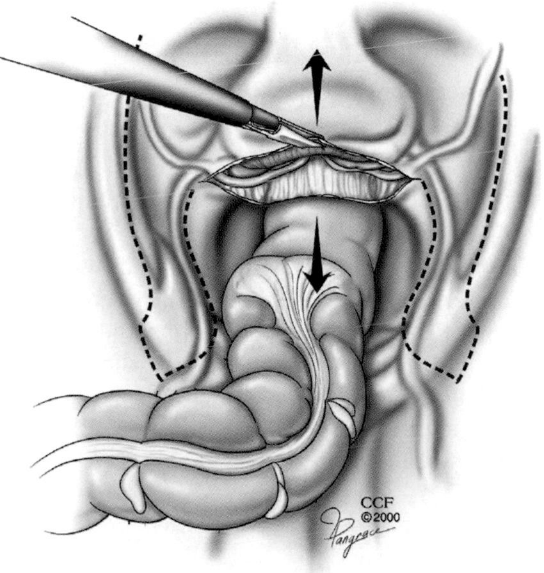

FIGURE 10.2. The peritoneum of the anterior aspect of the pouch of Douglas is incised to directly expose Denonvilliers' fascia, which is then incised transversely to expose the anterior aspect of the rectum

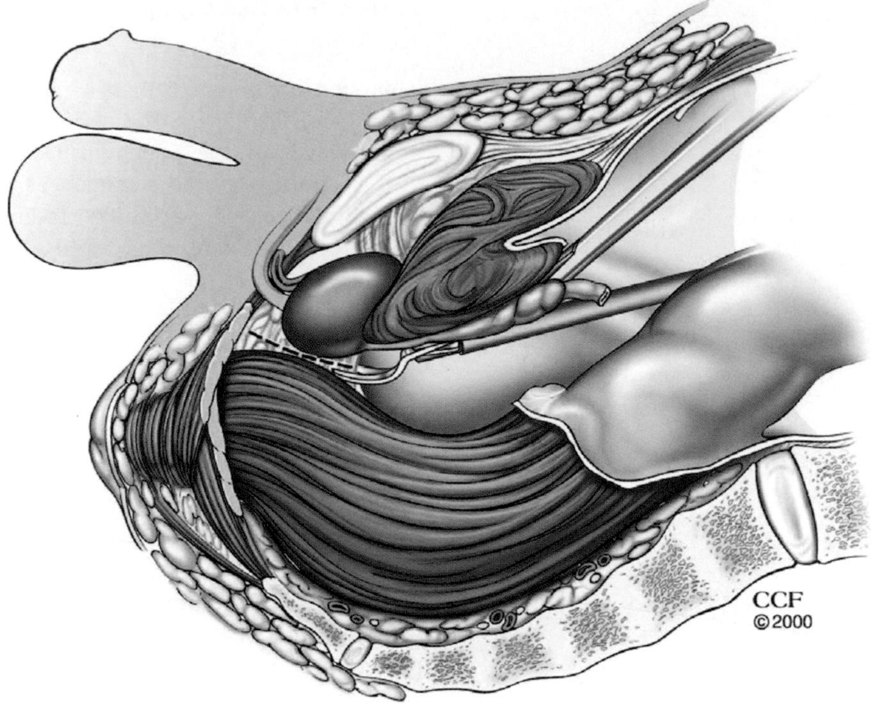

FIGURE 10.3. The dissection is continued toward the apex of the prostate to facilitate further mobilization of the rectum and exposure of the bladder pedicles. Caution should be taken during this step, because the angle of dissection is not always optimal, and blind dissection could lead to rectal injury

greatly facilitates identification of the lateral aspect of the vesicoprostatic pedicles.

Dissection of the Ureters

The ureters are initially approached and dissected at the crossing over the common iliac artery and then further down to the bladder wall, with care to preserve their vascular supply. The ureters are clipped distally with locking clips and divided, and the distal ureteral margins are sent for histopathology if indicated. The dissected distal ureters are then positioned above the level of the iliac vessels.

Transection of the Vesical and Prostatic Pedicles

After the rectum has been completely mobilized and the bladder laterally dissected off the pelvic wall, the vascular pedicles of the bladder and the prostate will already be well defined.

Leaving the bladder attached to the anterior abdominal wall by the two medial and the median umbilical ligaments is important to facilitate exposure of the vascular pedicles. The vascular pedicles of the bladder and prostate are divided using laparoscopic vascular staplers (to save time). The stapler may need to be reloaded three or four times to completely divide the pedicle on each side (Figure 10.5). Other instruments, depending on the surgeon's preference, can be used to safely transect the vascular pedicles of the bladder.

Mobilization of the Bladder and Dissection of the Urethra

The approach of the Retzius space is similar to that in radical prostatectomy (see Chapter 9), but the medial umbilical ligaments and urachus are incised much higher on the abdominal wall before the Retzius space is developed. The bladder is then dissected off the abdominal wall, and the anterior

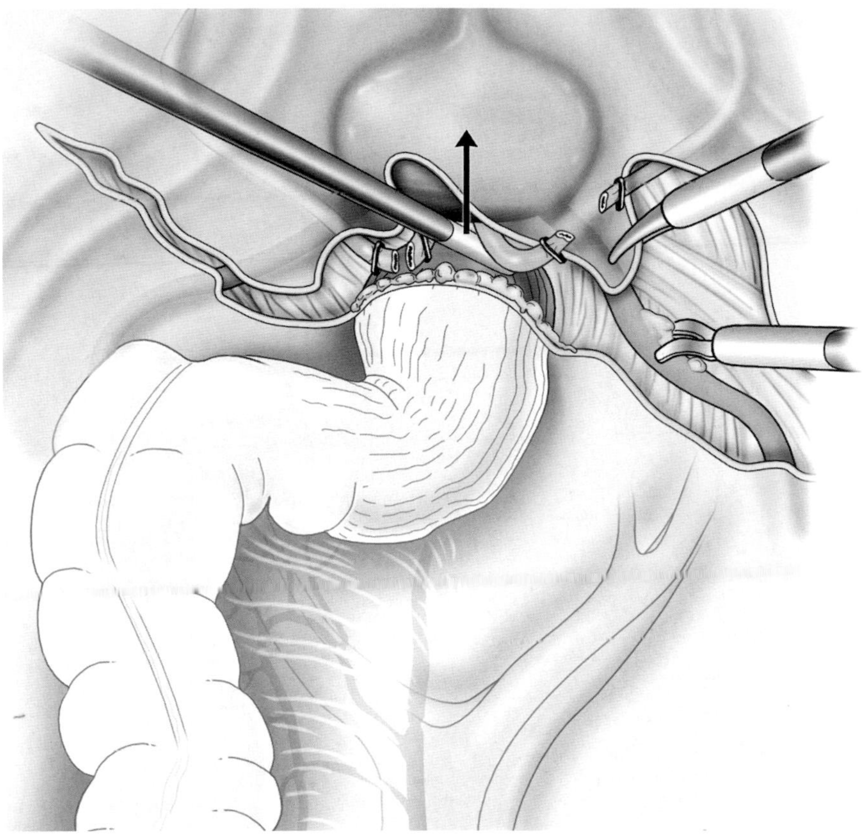

FIGURE 10.4. The anterior pelvic peritoneum is incised laterally on both sides, along the common iliac artery and then anteriorly lateral to the medial umbilical ligaments. The vas deferens are transected at this level. This dissection exposes the ureters medial to the umbilical ligaments. The ureters are dissected toward the bladder, clipped, and then transected

aspect of the prostate with the endopelvic fascia is exposed. The incision of the endopelvic fascia is completed toward the pubovesical ligaments. The ligaments are sharply divided to expose the apex of the prostate and the dorsal vascular complex. Once the membranous urethra and the dorsal vascular complex are exposed, the complex is ligated with suture material (e.g., Vicryl 2-0 on an SH needle) and then divided. The urethra and the apex of the prostate are fully dissected. The transection of the urethra depends on the planned urinary diversion and varies from full urethral preservation (for orthotopic neobladder) to complete urethral resection at the level of the pelvic floor muscle (for supravesical urinary diversion). After transection, the prostatic urethra must be closed immediately at the prostatic apex to avoid urine spillage in the peritoneal cavity. The closure is performed with Vicryl 2-0 suture in a figure-8 pattern.

The rectourethralis muscle is divided, completing the radical cystoprostatectomy. The specimen is immediately placed in an endoscopic bag and positioned in the upper abdomen.

Specimen Retrieval

In male patients, the method of the bladder retrieval depends on the planned urinary diversion. If the sigma-rectum pouch (Mainz Pouch II) is planned, the opened rectum offers an advantageous way to remove the specimen in an endoscopic bag via the anal canal. If the ileal loop is the proposed urinary diversion, an incision (4-5 cm) is made at the level of the previously selected stoma site (usually at the

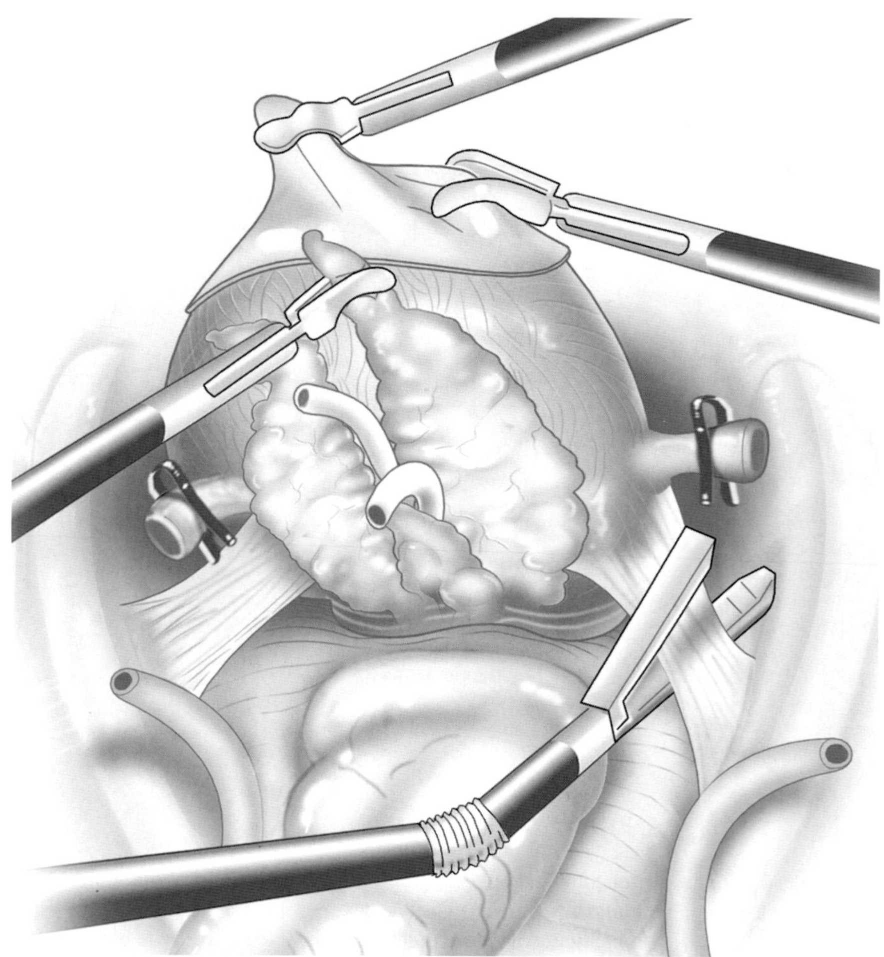

FIGURE 10.5. After the bladder pedicle has been dissected and clearly identified, it can be transected safely with an endoscopic stapler. In all other situations, individual ligation of the vascular pedicles is preferred

right pararectal region) to retrieve the bladder. If an orthotopic neobladder is planned, an infraumbilical incision (4-5 cm) at the midline is most appropriate for removal of the specimen.

Anterior Exenteration in Women

The technique of laparoscopic radical cystectomy is somewhat different in women than in men. The female patient is placed in the lithotomy position to allow access to the vagina, which is packed with a vaginal patch.

Peritoneal access is established the same as in male patients. The bladder, uterus, and ovaries are more easily handled if these organs are fixed together en bloc.

Suture of the Uterine Fundus and Bladder

After the abdominal cavity has been carefully inspected, the ovaries are identified. The infundibulopelvic ligaments are exposed by incising the overlying peritoneum, and then divided between locking clips. The broad ligaments are incised bilaterally, parallel to the fallopian tubes, rendering the tubo-ovarian complex completely free. The excision of the anterior pelvic organs en bloc is facilitated by suturing the bladder, the uterine fundus, and the ovaries together. After this maneuver, the assistant can easily retract the uterus anteriorly.

Mobilization of the rectum off the posterior vaginal wall, lateral bladder mobilization, and transection of the bladder pedicles are similar to the techniques in men.

Dissection of the Bladder Neck and Proximal Urethra

The dissection begins with a bilateral incision of the endopelvic fascia, which exposes the pubovesical ligaments and the bladder neck. The ligaments are sharply divided to expose the dorsal vascular complex, which is divided after ligation using Vicryl 2-0 on an SH needle (see Chapter 9, Radical Prostatectomy). Transection of the dorsal vascular complex exposes the membranous urethra, which is then transected at the level of the pelvic floor. The vesical side of the urethra is immediately closed to avoid any urine spillage in the peritoneal cavity. The closure is performed with Vicryl 2-0 in a figure-8 pattern.

Grasping the suture, the surgeon retracts the bladder toward the peritoneal cavity and off the anterior vaginal wall as far as possible. A vaginal sponge facilitates identification of the vagina. At the level of the cervix, the anterior vaginal wall is divided, and the vaginal sponge removed.

At this point, the vagina is open and the first assistant must press a sterile sponge stick against the introitus to avoid extensive gas loss.

After the posterior vaginal wall has been transected, the specimen is completely mobilized and can be extracted; the assistant introduces a 15-mm endoscopic bag through the open vagina into the pelvis. The specimen is entrapped in the bag, which is closed and then removed through the vagina. The vagina is then closed with Vicryl 2-0 suture on an SH needle.

Bilateral Pelvic Lympth Node Dissection

See Chapter 8 (Pelvic Lymph Node Dissection) for a detailed description of this technique. Extended pelvic lymph node dissection is most easily performed after the bladder has been removed from the pelvis and the ureters have been mobilized and moved away from the iliac vessels. An extended bilateral pelvic lymph node dissection can then be performed safely. The usual limits of the dissection are the pubic bone caudally, the aortic bifurcation cranially, the genitofemoral nerve anteriorly, and the internal iliac artery posteriorly.

The lymph nodes are removed in separate packets in an endoscopic bag.

Urinary Diversion

Radical cystectomy involves only a few additional simple steps beyond those required for laparoscopic radical prostatectomy. These include dissecting the ureters and transecting the lateral vesical pedicles with laparoscopic staplers. However, urinary diversion remains a technical challenge when performed laparoscopically. Except for the Mainz pouch II, performing the diversion through an abdominal incision, pulling out the neobladder and the ureters, is recommended. The laparotomy approach provides good functional results with the neobladder or the ileal loop conduit and significantly decreases the morbidity and surgical time as compared with a urinary diversion performed laparoscopically. The laparotomy approach still provides the benefits of a minimally invasive approach, because the abdominal incision is reduced in length and stretch and the duration of intraperitoneal exposure is shortened.

Laparoscopic Ileal Loop: Extracorporeal

The ileal loop urinary diversion has been a standard type of urinary diversion for many years. Although urinary diversion by ileal conduit can be performed by laparoscopy alone, performing a laparotomy after the laparoscopic cystectomy is recommended to extract the specimen and to construct the ileal conduit urinary diversion.

Marking the Ureters

Before the specimen is removed during laparotomy, the ureters are marked with holding sutures of different colors (white/blue, Vicryl 4-0). These markings are helpful in two later steps, viz, crossing the left ureter underneath the sigmoid colon and identifying the ureters during the laparotomy, especially in obese patients.

The distal 5-6 cm of the left ureter is dissected with care to preserve the periureteral tissue and its vascular supply. A space is bluntly created just anterior to the sacrum and posterior to the mesentery of the sigmoid colon to allow the passage of the left ureter to the right using the previously placed holding suture. Both holding sutures are placed extracorporeally and secured with a clamp just before the specimen is removed.

Ileal Loop

The mini-laparotomy (a 3-4 cm extension of the right side 10-mm pararectal port) is used for specimen removal. The distal ileum is identified and brought in front of the abdominal wall. A small-bowel segment, 12-15 cm long, is isolated with an intestinal stapler. The continuity of the bowel is reestablished by a functional end-to-end anastomosis using intestinal staplers. The mesentery is reapproximated using absorbable sutures, and the distal ileum relocated in the abdomen. The distal ureters are brought in the operative field and properly aligned using the different-colored holding sutures. The spatulated ureters are stented and anastomosed in Bricker fashion to the ileal loop using Monocryl 4-0 sutures. Eventually, double-J stents can be used to drain the kidneys if there is any doubt regarding the quality of the ureteroileal anastomosis. The proximal end of the conduit is replaced in the abdomen. The fascia of the rectus muscle is partially closed, leaving only enough space to allow passage of the conduit. The loop is secured to the muscle fascia, and the stoma is matured.

Laparoscopic Control

Pneumoperitoneum is reestablished, and the proper placement of the ileal loop confirmed. The loop is brought retroperitoneal and sutured (Vicryl 2-0) to the anterolateral abdominal wall to prevent potential internal hernia.

A Jackson-Pratt drain is left in the pelvis. The fascia of the 10-mm port sites is closed under direct visualization with Vicryl 0 suture. The pneumoperitoneum is drained, and the procedure completed.

Postoperative Care

The Jackson-Pratt drain is removed as drainage decreases and the absence of any urine leak is confirmed by determining whether the drainage fluid contains creatinine. The nasogastric tube is removed the first day after surgery, with the patient resuming liquid intake. Oral intake of solid food can begin 3 days after surgery depending on the clinical situation.

The patient is usually discharged between 6 and 8 days after surgery. If double-J stents have been used, they should be removed in 2-3 weeks.

Laparoscopic Mainz Pouch II: Intracorporeal

The Mainz pouch II (sigma-rectum) is a modification of a ureterosigmoidostomy. The sigma-rectum pouch has two prominent benefits: it is relatively easy to construct and it allows excellent 24-hour continence in properly selected patients. In men, the sigma-rectum pouch has an additional benefit in that the opening of the sigmoid and rectum can be used to extract the specimen without the need for an abdominal incision.

Preoperative Evaluation

Before surgery, the patient undergoes outpatient sigmoidoscopy to exclude diverticulosis and tumors in the rectum-sigmoid area. Further selection criteria include a competent anal sphincter (assessed by the ability to hold a 200-300 mL water enema for 2 hours) and adequate renal function (serum creatinine <1.5 mg/dL).

Operative Technique

Preparation of the Rectum: An antimesenteric enterotomy is created at the rectosigmoid junction and extended 10 cm proximally and 10 cm distally (Figure 10.6). In men, this allows for transanal removal of the specimen. The posterior walls of the rectum and sigmoid are then anastomosed side-to-side with a running monofilament absorbable 3-0 suture to form the posterior wall of the pouch (Figure 10.7).

Ureteral Anastomosis: Non-refluxing ureteral anastomoses are formed by preparing a 3-4 cm submucosal bed in the posterior plate of the pouch, and then drawing the mobilized ureters through the pouch plate and securing with 3-4 sutures (Vicryl 4-0) in this previously formed bed. After 8F single-J ureteral catheters have been inserted (via the opened rectum), the submucosal tunnels are completed by suturing the mucosa over the ureters

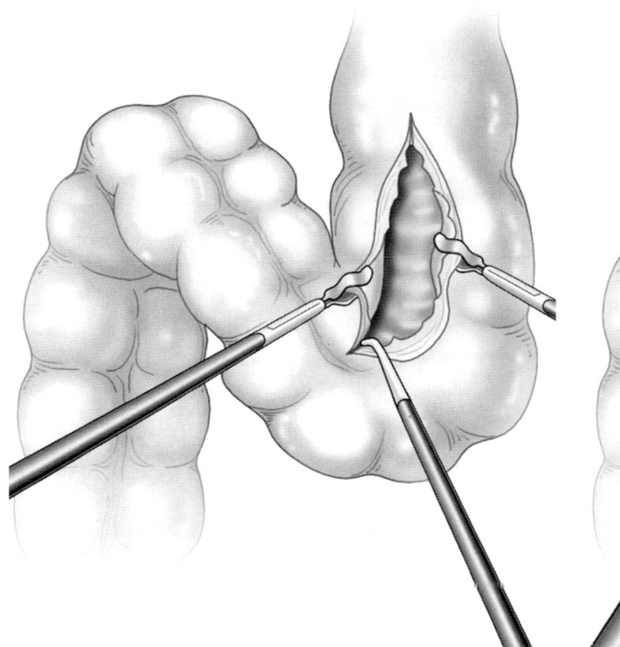

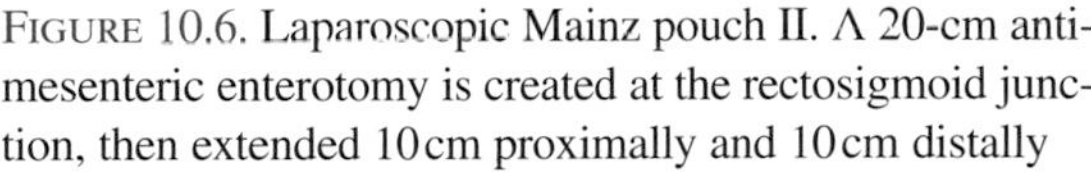

FIGURE 10.6. Laparoscopic Mainz pouch II. A 20-cm antimesenteric enterotomy is created at the rectosigmoid junction, then extended 10cm proximally and 10cm distally

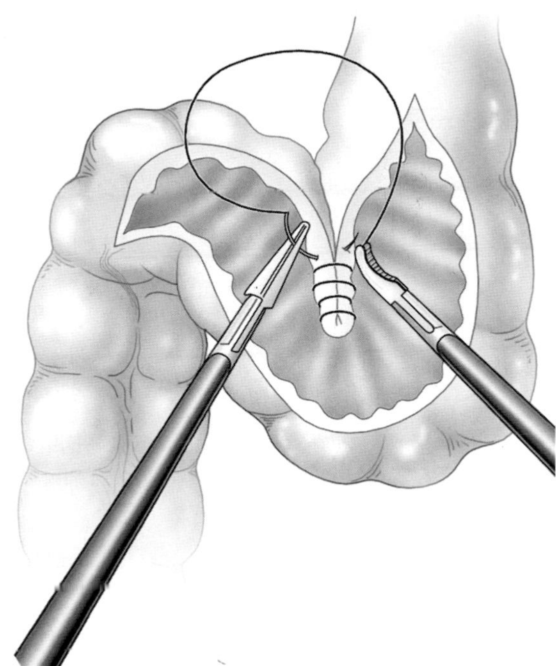

FIGURE 10.7. Creation of the posterior plate of the Mainz pouch II, suturing side-to-side the posterior walls of the rectum and the sigmoid colon using absorbable monofilament 3-0

(Vicryl 4-0) (Figure 10.8). The ureteral single-J stents are brought out of the anus, and the pouch is drained with a transanal 26F Nelaton catheter. The anterior wall of the pouch is closed with a running 3-0 Maxon suture (Figure 10.9).

Completion of the Procedure: The pelvis is drained with a single Jackson-Pratt drain through one of the lateral 5-mm trocar incisions. The fascia of the 10-mm port sites is closed under direct vision with Vicryl 0. The pneumoperitoneum is drained and the procedure completed. The Nelaton catheter as well as both single-J stents are fixed with sutures to the skin close to the anus.

Postoperative Care: The Jackson-Pratt drain is removed as drainage decreases and the absence of urine leakage is confirmed by determining whether the drainage fluid contains creatinine. The nasogastric tube is removed the day after surgery. The patient can resume liquid intake 2 days after surgery and intake of solid food 3-4 days after surgery depending on the clinical situation. The ureteral stents are removed 7 days after surgery; and the pouch catheter 8 days after surgery, when the patient is discharged from the hospital.

Ileal Neobladder (Studer): Extra- and Intracorporeal

Despite the simplicity of the Mainz pouch II and the good quality of life it provides, the orthotopic neobladder remains the gold standard for urinary diversion in patients undergoing radical cystectomy. A purely laparoscopic procedure, even if technically possible, should not be performed at this time; instead, a laparoscopic-assisted technique for building an orthotopic neobladder is recommended. A practical advantage is that the abdominal incision needed for specimen removal can be used to create the neobladder outside of the abdomen. Once completed, the neobladder is then introduced into the pelvis, the abdominal incision closed, and the abdomen re-insufflated. Then, a laparoscopic approach is used for the anastomosis between the urethra and the neobladder, and for

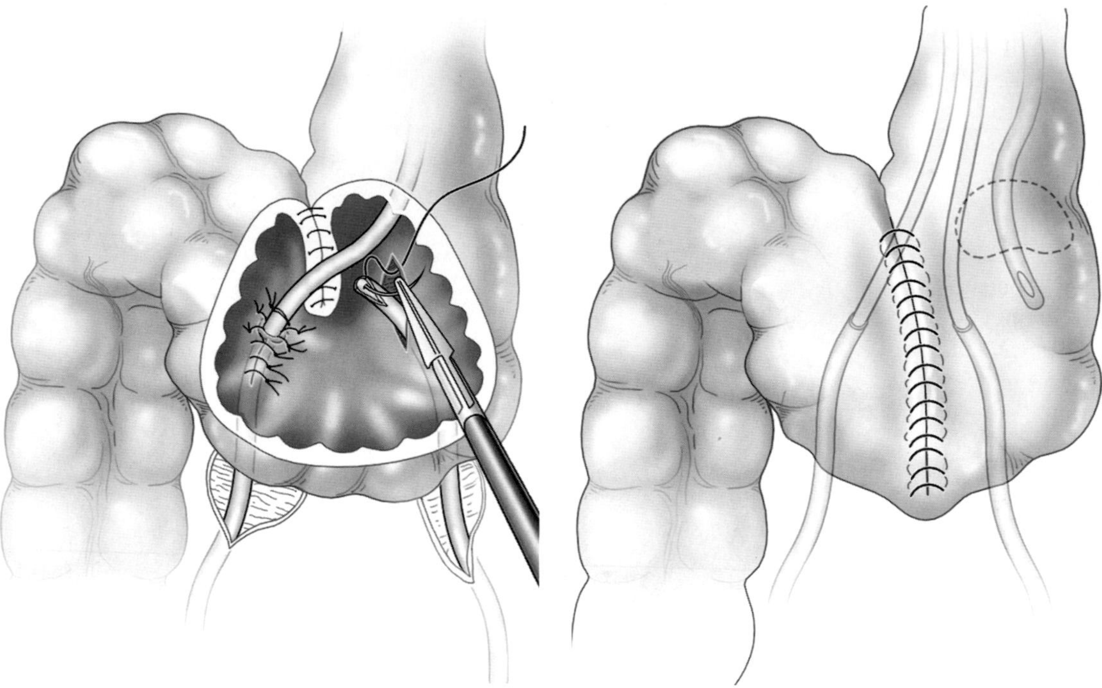

FIGURE 10.8. Antireflux implantation of the ureters on the posterior plate of the pouch using a submucosal incision that is subsequently reapproximated over the ureters

FIGURE 10.9. Completed Mainz pouch II: the two ureteral single-J stents are brought out of the anus, and the pouch is drained with a transanal 26F Nelaton catheter. The pouch is closed with a running suture of 3-0 absorbable monofilament

the two anastomoses between the neobladder and the ureters.

Marking the Ureters

As in the creation of an ileal loop, in the ileal neobladder procedure, the ureters must be marked. Before performing the mini-laparotomy for specimen removal, the left ureter is crossed underneath the sigmoid colon toward the right side and both ureters are marked with holding sutures of different colors.

Creating the Reservoir

The incision for removal of the bladder should be located at the midline subumbilical incision (a 4-cm extension of the subumbilical 10-mm trocar). Thc distal ileum is brought out through this incision, and 60 cm of ileum is isolated, preserving the last ileal loop and the ileocecal junction.

Vascularization of the bowel segment is preserved using the standard transillumination technique. Isolation of the loop as well as side-to-side anastomosis of the distal ileum is performed using intestinal staplers. The window in the mesenterium should be closed with 4 or 5 interrupted stitches (Monocryl 3-0) to prevent an internal hernia.

The re-anastomosed distal ileum is replaced into the intraperitoneal cavity, while the isolated ileum segment remains extracorporeal. The distal 50 cm of the isolated ileum segment is detubularized along the antimesenteric line using the electrocautery blade. The proximal 10 cm of the isolated loop is maintained intact for the Studer limb. The detubularized part of the ileum is folded in a U shape, and the posterior plate of the neobladder is created with a running suture of the corresponding edges of the detubularized ileum using Monocryl 3-0. Starting from the chimney, the anterior wall of the pouch is closed with an running suture (Monocryl 3-0), except for the remaining opening at the most distal part intended to serve as the "bladder neck," which will be used for the anastomosis with the urethra. The almost completely fashioned neobladder is than carefully reinserted into the abdomen and the mini-laparotomy is closed, except for the opening of the subumbilical camera port.

Urethroileal Anastomosis

After the pneumoperitoneum has been reestablished, the remaining distal opening of the neobladder is identified and selected for the urethroileal anastomosis. Care must be taken to ensure that the mesenterium of the ileal neobladder is not under tension and that the mesenteric pedicle is not twisted.

The anastomosis is performed with interrupted or running sutures using Monocryl 3-0 on an RB-1 needle (similar to that in a laparoscopic radical prostatectomy, Figure 10.10). Fixing the neobladder to the urethra facilitates the subsequent ureterointestinal anastomosis.

Ureteroileal Anastomosis

The ureteroileal anastomosis is performed intracorporeally using free-hand laparoscopic suturing techniques.

After the Studer chimney has been identified, the left ureter is brought into the operative field, properly aligned regarding the length, and spatulated. After an ileotomy on the left side of the chimney, the left ureter (corner of spatulation) is fixed to the ileotomy with one stitch (Vicryl 4-0, RB-1 needle). A double-J stent (usually 26/7F) is delivered into the intraperitoneal cavity over the right lateral 5-mm port. The proximal loop of the stent is inserted into the ureter and advanced into the renal pelvis using a guide wire. The distal loop is inserted into the Studer chimney. The ureteroileal anastomosis is completed with two running sutures (Monocryl 4-0, RB-1 needle).

The right ureteroileal anastomosis is completed on the right side of the chimney in a similar manner. The constructed orthotopic ileal neobladder is irrigated through the Foley catheter to check for any leakage.

Completing the Procedure

After hemostasis has been confirmed, the pelvis is irrigated and cleaned, and a Jackson-Pratt drain inserted through the left lateral 5-mm port and

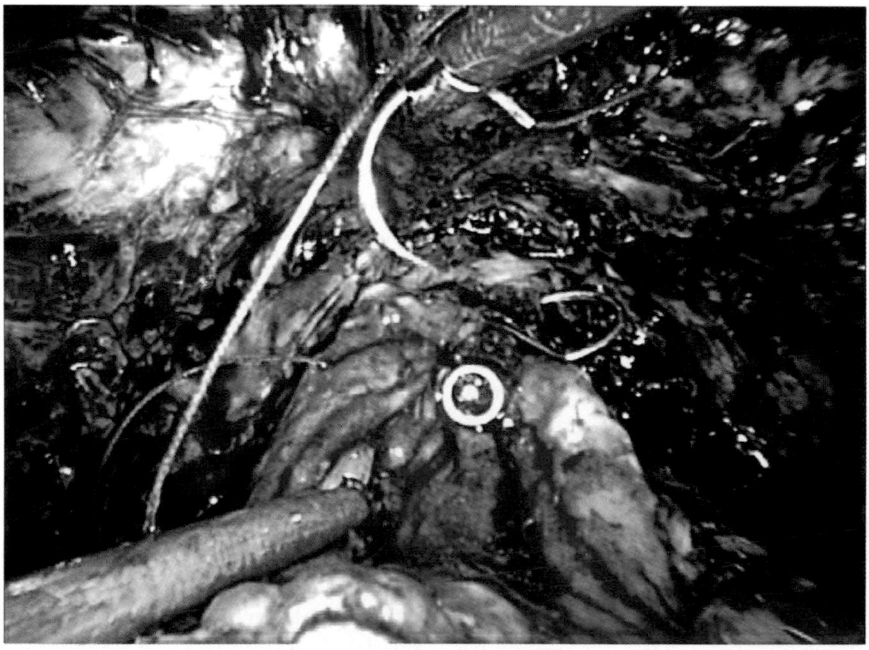

FIGURE 10.10. Laparoscopic anastomosis between the neobladder and the urethra, after the neobladder has been conventionally built. The neobladder is then positioned in the pelvis and the anastomosis is completed laparoscopically, which has the advantages of a smaller abdominal incision and a more accurate placement of the stitches

placed in the pelvis. All trocars are then removed, and the port site incisions closed as usual.

Postoperative Care

The urethral Foley catheter is irrigated every 4-6 hours for the first 3 days after surgery and 3-4 times a day thereafter. The Jackson-Pratt drain is removed as drainage decreases and the absence of any urine leak is confirmed by determining whether the draining fluid contains creatinine.

The nasogastric tube is removed the first day after surgery. The patient resumes liquid intake 2 days after surgery and intake of solid food 3 days after surgery depending on the clinical situation.

The patient is discharged from the hospital 5-6 days after surgery, with the Foley catheter and both double-J stents in place. A cystoscopy is performed 14 days after surgery as an outpatient procedure to remove the ureteral stents, and the catheter is removed 21 days after surgery after a cystogram reveals no leakage of the neobladder.

Complications

Intraoperative Complications

Iliac Vessel Injury

During the lateral bladder dissection and during the lymph node dissection, the potential for injury of the external iliac artery or vein is real. Injuries are more problematic in the external iliac artery than in the vein. The use of monopolar current close to the vessels has a particularly high potential for injury. The first maneuver in the event of an injury of the iliac external vein or artery is compression with a peanut grasper. Increasing the pneumoperitoneum up to 20 mm Hg will help control venous bleeding; however, arterial bleeding will continue. When possible, any attempt should be made to dissect the injured vessel proximal and caudal to the injury while the assistant maintains pressure on the site of injury. The goal is to create enough space proximal and distal to the injury to place atraumatic raged graspers to control the bleeding. Sometimes, an additional trocar must be inserted to allow proper placement of the graspers. After the vessel has been clamped distal and proximal to the defect, the injury can be inspected and sutured with Prolene 3-0 or 4-0. Prolene 4-0 suture, approximately 4 cm long and secured on one end with a locking clip, is recommended. After the vessel hole has been closed with a running suture, an additional locking clip can hold the suture in place, avoiding the need to tie a knot.

When, however, the bleeding situation cannot be controlled by these techniques, the surgeon should not hesitate to convert to open surgery.

Bleeding from the Bladder Pedicle

Although rare, bleeding from the transected bladder pedicle can potentially occur. Veins of large size, when present, are particularly likely to be the cause of such bleeding. Again, the first measures to control the bleeding are to increase the pneumoperitoneum up to 20 mm Hg and to compress the bleeding site with a peanut grasper. If stapler clips are in place (after use of laparoscopic stapler) or if the vein stump is retracted, use of bipolar forceps is unlikely to control the bleeding. The bleeding should be controlled by placing a figure-8 stitch with Monocryl 2-0 suture. Again, using a piece of suture 3-4 cm long, followed by use of a locking clip, is recommended.

Rectal Injury

As during laparoscopic radical prostatectomy, the potential for rectal injury during radical cystectomy increases with significant periprostatic fibrosis after severe inflammation or because of extensive cancer growth. If the rectum injury is recognized, the tear should be meticulously repaired. The edges are inspected, and a two-layer closure with Monocryl 3-0 suture (SH needle) is performed.

When necessary, an omental flap can be raised, transposed into the pelvis, and sutured over the repair for additional safety. A diverting colostomy is usually not necessary.

Postoperative Complications

Urine Leak

A high fluid output of the drain may indicate a leak of the ureteroileal anastomosis, the conduit, or the neobladder closure. The diagnosis can be confirmed by determining the presence of creatinine in the draining fluid.

In nearly all cases, the urine leak can be managed conservatively, and the leak will stop spontaneously at some point. However, in severe leaks, the urine drainage may need to be improved, and a temporary percutaneous nephrostomy diversion might be necessary for successful management.

Ileus

Prolonged paralytic ileus is a common postoperative problem after radical cystectomy and urinary diversion. The laparoscopic approach appears to decreases the incidence of this complication, probably because of the decreased bowel manipulation. Paralytic ileus usually resolves quickly with nasogastric decompression. If the ileus does not resolve within a few days, a diagnostic evaluation for bowel obstruction or peritonitis is warranted.

Appendix: Abbreviations

A aorta
Ad adrenal mass
AG adrenal gland
APA accessory pudendal artery
AV adrenal vein
AW abdominal wall

B bladder
BN bladder neck

C colon
CD descending colon
Ce cecum
CF colonic flexure
CIA common iliac artery
CIV common iliac vein
CS sigmoid colon
CT transverse colon
Cx cervix

D duodenum
DF Denonvilliers' fascia
Di diaphragm
DJL Treitz's ligament (duodenojejunic ligament)
DVC deep vascular complex

EPF endopelvic fascia
EIA external iliac artery
EIV external iliac vein

FT fallopian tube

G Gerota's fascia
GB gallbladder
GFN genitofemoral nerve
GPT gluteopudendal trunk
GV gonadal vessel

HDL hepatoduodenal ligament

IEA inferior epigastric artery
IEV inferior epigastric vein
IIA internal iliac artery
IMV inferior mesenteric vein
IO inguinal orifice
IPL infundibulopelvic ligament
IVC inferior vena cava

K kidney

L liver
LA levator ani muscle
LNP lymph node package
LUL lateral umbilical ligament
LV lumbar vein

MC mesocolon
MU membranous urethra
MUL medial umbilical ligament

NVB neurovascular bundle

O ovary
OA obturator artery
OIM obturator internus muscle
OM obturator muscle
ON obturator nerve

P prostate
PA prostatic apex
PC prostatic capsule
PCL phrenocolonic ligament
Pe peritoneum
PF prostatic fascia
PLL phrenicolienal ligament
PM psoas muscle
Pn pancreas
PP prostatic pedicle
PPF periprostatic fascia
PPL puboprostatic ligament
PS pubic symphysis
PUF periurethral fascia

R rectum
RA renal artery
RH renal hilum
RL round ligament
RMS rhabdomyosphincter
RP renal pelvis
RV renal vein

S spleen
SC spermatic cord
SDV superficial dorsal vein
SGA superior gluteal artery
Si sigmoid colon
SL splenocolic ligaments
SpV spermatic vessels
SU sphincteric urethra
SV seminal vesicles
SVA superior vesicle artery

TA tendinous arch of levator ani muscle
TF Toldt's fascia
TL line of Toldt

U ureter
Uh urethra
UL median umbilical ligament
US ultrasound probe
USL utero-sacral ligament
Ut uterus

V vas deferens
VC vena cava
VPM vesicoprostatic muscle

Index

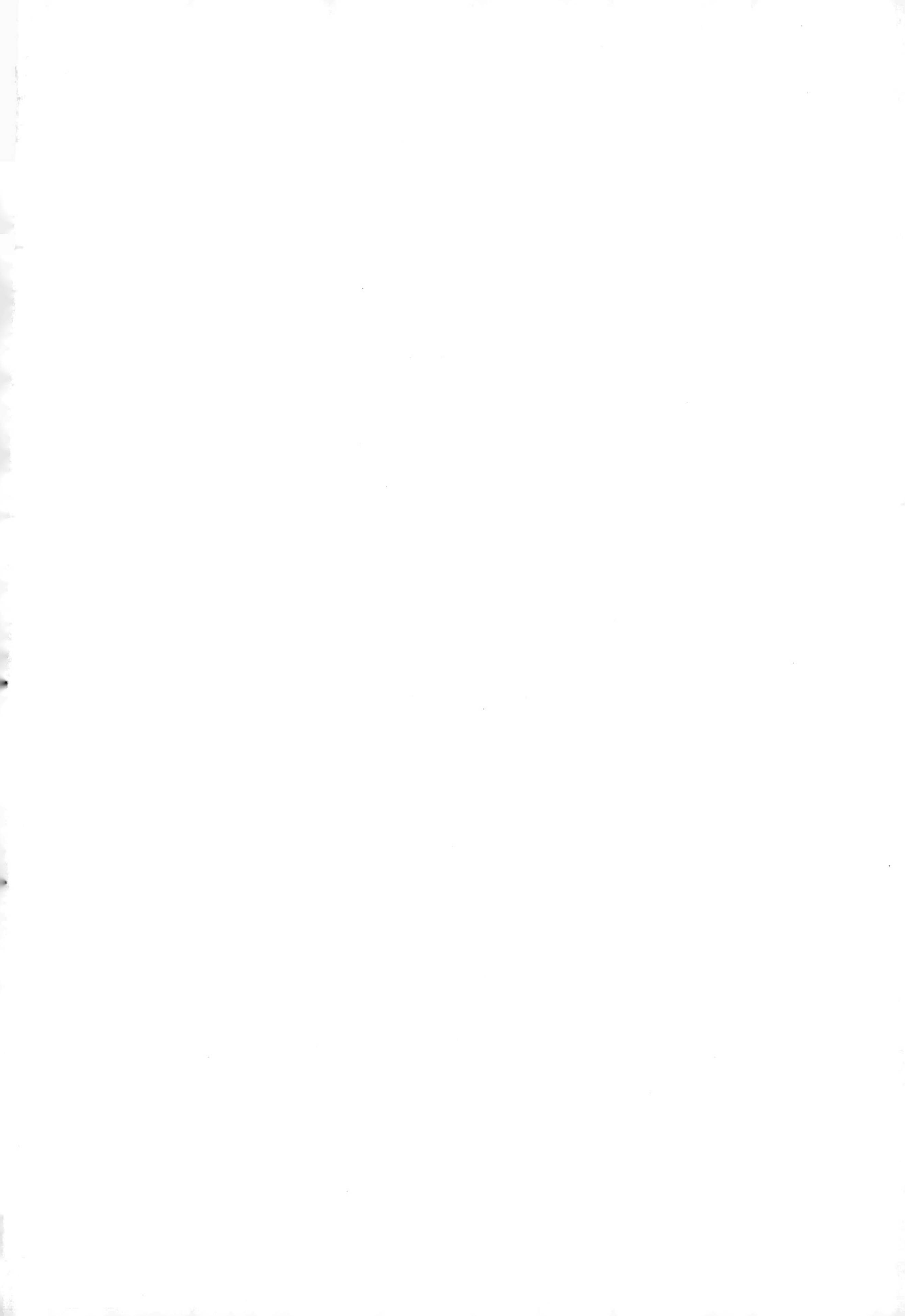